SHOULDER ARTHROSCOPY

EDITED BY

THEODORE A. BLAINE, MD
ASSOCIATE PROFESSOR OF ORTHOPAEDIC SURGERY
COLUMBIA UNIVERSITY
NEW YORK, NEW YORK

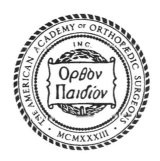

American Academy of Orthopaedic Surgeons

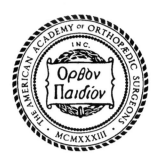

Shoulder Arthroscopy

Published 2006 by the
American Academy of Orthopaedic Surgeons
6300 North River Road
Rosemont, IL 60018
1-800-626-6726

The material presented in *Shoulder Arthroscopy* has been made available by the American Academy of Orthopaedic Surgeons for educational purposes only. This material is not intended to present the only, or necessarily best, methods or procedures for the medical situations discussed, but rather is intended to represent an approach, view, statement, or opinion of the author(s) or producer(s), which may be helpful to others who face similar situations.

Some drugs or medical devices demonstrated in Academy courses or described in Academy print or electronic publications have not been cleared by the Food and Drug Administration (FDA) or have been cleared for specific uses only. The FDA has stated that it is the responsibility of the physician to determine the FDA clearance status of each drug or device he or she wishes to use in clinical practice.

Furthermore, any statements about commercial products are solely the opinion(s) of the author(s) and do not represent an Academy endorsement or evaluation of these products. These statements may not be used in advertising or for any commercial purpose.

Some of the authors or the departments with which they are affiliated have received something of value from a commercial or other party related directly or indirectly to the subject of their chapter.

First Edition
Copyright © 2006 by the
American Academy of
Orthopaedic Surgeons

ISBN 10: 0-89203-412-2
ISBN 13: 978-0-89203-412-3

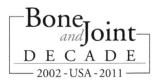

CONTRIBUTORS

Christopher S. Ahmad, MD
Assistant Professor of Orthopaedic Surgery
Department of Orthopaedic Surgery
New York Presbyterian Hospital
New York, New York

Sean F. Bak, MD
Fellow, The Shoulder Service
Department of Orthopaedic Surgery
Columbia-Presbyterian Medical Center
New York, New York

Louis U. Bigliani, MD
Frank E. Stinchfield Professor and Chairman
Department of Orthopaedic Surgery
Columbia University
New York, New York

Theodore A. Blaine, MD
Associate Professor of Orthopaedic Surgery
Columbia University
New York, New York

Patrick M. Connor, MD
OrthoCarolina
Charlotte, North Carolina

Donald F. D'Alessandro, MD
Chief, Sports Medicine and Shoulder Service
Carolinas Medical Center
Charlotte, North Carolina

Neal S. ElAttrache, MD
Director, Sports Medicine Fellowship
Kerlan-Jobe Orthopaedic Clinic
Los Angeles, California

Leesa M. Galatz, MD
Assistant Professor
Department of Orthopaedic Surgery
Washington University School of Medicine
St. Louis, Missouri

Charles L. Getz, MD
Assistant Professor
Department of Orthopaedic Surgery
University of Pennsylvania
Philadelphia, Pennsylvania

David L. Glaser, MD
Cali Family Assistant Professor of
  Orthopaedic Surgery
University of Pennsylvania
Philadelphia, Pennsylvania

Steven S. Goldberg, MD
Clinical Fellow
Department of Orthopaedic Surgery
Columbia University
New York, New York

Gregory D. Gramstad, MD
Fellow, Shoulder and Elbow Surgery
Department of Orthopaedic Surgery
Washington University School of Medicine
St. Louis, Missouri

Marshall A. Kuremsky, MD
Resident
Department of Orthopaedic Surgery
Carolinas Medical Center
Charlotte, North Carolina

Contributors (cont.)

William N. Levine, MD
Vice Chairman and Associate Professor
Department of Orthopaedic Surgery
Columbia University
New York, New York

Seth R. Miller, MD
Assistant in Orthopaedic Surgeery
Columbia-Presbyterian Medical Center
New York, New York

Matthew L. Ramsey, MD
Assistant Professor of Orthopedic Surgery
Shoulder and Elbow Service
Penn Orthopedic Institute
University of Pennsylvania
Philadelphia, Pennsylvania

Gerald R. Williams, Jr, MD
Professor, Chief of Orthopaedic Surgery
Penn-Presbyterian Medical Center
University of Pennsylvania
Philadelphia, Pennsylvania

Ken Yamaguchi, MD
Professor of Orthopaedic Surgery
Chief, Shoulder and Elbow Service
Department of Orthopaedic Surgery
Washington University School of Medicine
St. Louis, Missouri

CONTENTS

PREFACE

O ver the past decade, there has been a tremendous increase in the indications for and uses of arthroscopy in the diagnosis and treatment of shoulder disorders. This increase has produced a multitude of new instruments, implants, and techniques. This monograph provides a concise yet complete overview of the most common diagnoses and procedures for which shoulder arthroscopy currently is used. Following an opening chapter that discusses basic anatomy, arthroscopy set-up, and surgical techniques, subsequent chapters discuss basic and advanced arthroscopic treatment of rotator cuff disease, instability, labral and biceps lesions, adhesive capsulitis, and arthritis. The final chapter provides an excellent discussion of the complications of shoulder arthroscopy, which is an important resource for all surgeons performing arthroscopic shoulder surgery. The authors have emphasized principles, indications, and techniques, and I hope that this information will be useful to shoulder surgeons, arthroscopists, sports medicine physicians, and general orthopaedists alike.

A group of expert arthroscopic shoulder surgeons were assembled to produce this monograph, and I am greatly indebted to them for their time, effort, and enthusiasm in sharing their expertise. I owe a particular debt of gratitude to my mentor, chairman, and friend, Dr. Louis Bigliani, for inspiring my passion for shoulder surgery and for his unwavering support. Additionally, I would like to acknowledge the outstanding efforts, patience, and perseverance of the AAOS publications staff, with a special thanks to Joan Abern, for the production of this monograph. Finally, I would like to take this opportunity to thank my amazing wife, Danielle, and our wonderful children, Logan, Gabrielle, Luke, and Sophia. While prioritizing the various responsibilities of a career in orthopaedic surgery is a continual challenge, I am so fortunate to have a wife and family whose constant love makes these decisions easy for me.

Theodore A. Blaine, MD
Editor

CHAPTER 1

ARTHROSCOPIC SHOULDER ANATOMY

GREGORY D. GRAMSTAD, MD
LEESA M. GALATZ, MD
KEN YAMAGUCHI, MD

Mastery of the arthroscopic anatomy of the shoulder is essential to avoiding complications and treatment failures and to performing successful arthroscopic surgery. This chapter presents arthroscopic shoulder anatomy and its important variations, beginning with a review of requisite superficial anatomy as it relates to portal placement and continuing with a discussion of deep arthroscopic anatomy.

SUPERFICIAL ANATOMY AND PORTAL PLACEMENT

Appreciation of the palpable bony landmarks is essential to the creation of safe, accurate, and reproducible portals. The acromion, scapular spine, distal clavicle, acromioclavicular (AC) joint, and coracoid tip are all used to locate the placement of key portals. Three points greatly facilitate the correct identification of the superficial landmarks: the anterolateral and posterolateral corners of the acromion and the supraclavicular fossa at the confluence of the posterior distal clavicle and the anterior scapular spine (Neviaser portal). The posterolateral corner of the acromion is the most easily identifiable landmark, even in overweight individuals, and should be identified first. The anterolateral corner is more difficult to palpate secondary to the underlying greater tuberosity; however, knowing that it is in line with the anterior distal clavicle helps identify this point. The supraclavicular fossa is quite easily palpated in most individuals and represents the posterior aspect of the

FIGURE 1

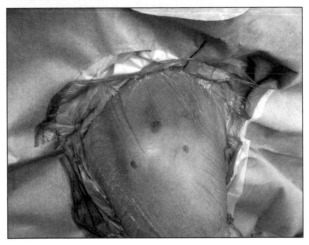

Marking the topographic anatomy is an important first step in the accurate creation of portals. The posterolateral corner and the supraclavicular fossa usually are palpated easily. In contrast, the anterolateral corner of the acromion can be difficult to locate, especially in large shoulders. The three points will usually form the apices of an equilateral triangle.

AC joint that is just anterior to the Neviaser supraclavicular portal.[1] When appropriately marked, these points almost always approximate the tips of an equilateral triangle (Figure 1). The lateral acromion, distal clavicle, scapular spine, AC joint, and coracoid tip are then outlined to complete the orientation. The location of the coracoid tip is important for anterior portal placement, but it can be difficult to palpate in overweight individ-

FIGURE 2

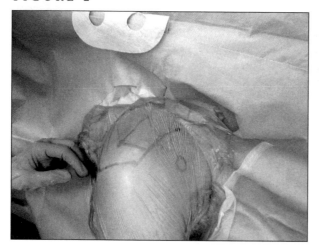

Using the triangle as a foundation, the remaining anatomy is marked. It is helpful to remember that the AC joint lies anterior to the supraclavicular fossa and that the coracoid tip lies in the approximate center of the arc formed by the distal clavicle.

FIGURE 3

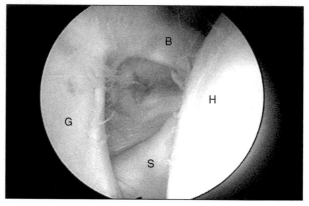

Arthroscopic image of the right shoulder with the patient in the beach chair position. The rotator interval triangle should be visualized when using the outside-in technique for creation of the standard anterior portal. Arthroscopically, the interval triangle is defined medially by the anterior glenoid (G), superiorly by the anterior supraspinatus, usually obscured by the intra-articular long head of the biceps tendon (B), and inferiorly by the rolled superior border of the subscapularis tendon (S). H = humeral head.

uals. If the anterior margin of the distal clavicle is viewed as an arc, the coracoid tip resides in its approximate center (Figure 2).

The posterior portal is often established first as the viewing portal. Its standard location is 2 to 3 cm inferior and 1 to 2 cm medial to the posterolateral corner of the acromion. The axillary nerve is relatively safe in this location; it is reported to be an average of 5 cm from the posterolateral corner of the acromion, with a minimum distance of approximately 3 cm in short women.[2-4] If posteroinferior capsular surgery is likely to be required, the posterior portal should be made more lateral, directly inferior to the corner, to facilitate viewing and instrumentation of the posteroinferior capsule and labrum.[5] An accessory posterior portal placed up to 3 cm lateral and 5 cm inferior to the posterolateral corner can be established safely while maintaining a distance of 3 cm from the axillary nerve.[4] This portal may be required to improve the angle of approach for anchor placement on the posteroinferior glenoid. If the indirect technique for distal clavicle resection is planned, a slightly more medial than normal placement of the posterior portal can aid AC joint visualization.

Anterior portals are placed in the rotator interval. The interval is seen arthroscopically as a triangle defined medially by the glenoid, superiorly by the intra-articu-lar biceps tendon, and inferiorly by the rolled border of the subscapularis muscle (Figure 3). The exact location and number of anterior portals depends on the pathology discovered during the initial diagnostic arthroscopy. Care should be taken to place all portals lateral to the coracoid tip to avoid the brachial plexus and axillary vessels that lie medially. When only one portal is required, spinal needle localization and a simple outside-in technique often will be sufficient. When multiple anterior portals are required, precise capsular penetration of each portal should ensure an adequate working space within the confines of the rotator interval. This penetration can be accomplished with either an inside-out technique or an outside-in technique using cannulated portal dilators. One advantage to the outside-in technique is the ability to use the initial trochar as a guide to determine whether the proposed portal placement will permit an adequate angle of approach and access to the essential structures (Figure 4).

For anterior instability surgery, the anteroinferior portal should enter the glenohumeral joint as laterally as possible over the superior edge of the subscapularis. The anterosuperior portal will enter anterior to the supraspinatus, just behind the long head of the biceps tendon, so that the cannula can be directed either ante-

FIGURE 4

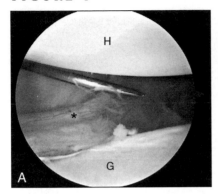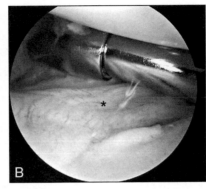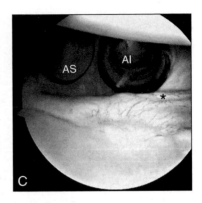

Arthroscopic images of the right shoulder with the patient in the lateral decubitus position. The middle glenohumeral ligament (asterisk) is easily visualized, whereas the anteroinferior glenoid labrum and anterior band of the inferior glenohumeral ligament have been avulsed and lie medial to the glenoid rim. **A,** A guidewire is used to accurately position the anteroinferior portal in the lateral rotator interval for Bankart repair. The ability to reach the inferior glenoid is verified before the portal is dilated **(B)**. **C,** Accurate cannulation of the anterosuperior (AS) and antero-inferior (AI) portals should permit the unobstructed use of instruments through either portal. Asterisk = midglenoid notch; H = humeral head; G = glenoid.

rior or posterior to the tendon. Externally, the two cannulas will be almost perpendicular to each other when properly positioned. This arrangement maximizes the working space between the portals both externally and within the joint. An anteroinferior, or 5 o'clock portal, that uses an inside-out technique and pierces the lower third of the subscapularis muscle has been described.[6] This portal generally is not necessary to reach the inferior capsule, and it has been reported to put the cephalic vein and humeral articular cartilage at risk.[4,7]

Superolateral portals have been established at almost every conceivable position from anterior to posterior along the lateral acromion. The key to customizing these portals is avoiding the humeral head and understanding axillary nerve anatomy. As the nerve traverses the undersurface of the deltoid from posterior to anterior, the distance from the lateral acromial edge increases slightly. The minimum safe distance has been shown to be 3 cm from the posterolateral corner and 4 cm at the AC joint with the arm adducted.[3] If these distances are respected, portals can be positioned to maximize the angle of approach to the essential pathologic structures while minimizing the risk of damage to the axillary nerve. Spinal needle localization should confirm precise portal position for arthroscopy of both the intra-articular and subacromial spaces.

LONG HEAD OF THE BICEPS TENDON

Diagnostic arthroscopy typically begins with identification of the long head of the biceps tendon and its origin at the superior glenoid. A high degree of normal anatomic variation exists at the biceps origin and the anterosuperior labrum. The long head of the biceps originates from the supraglenoid tubercle and the posterosuperior labrum. Habermeyer and associates[8] reported that 50% of cadaveric specimens had an entirely labral origin, 20% had an isolated origin from the supraglenoid tubercle, and the remaining 30% had a dual origin. Using histologic examination of 105 cadaveric shoulders, Vangsness and associates[9] determined that the biceps had a dual origin in 40% to 60% of specimens, with the rest originating from the labrum alone. They identified four variations of labral insertion: type I, the labral attachment is entirely posterior (22%); type II, most of the labral attachment is posterior, with some anterior component (33%); type III, equal anterior and posterior labral attachments (37%); and type IV, mostly anterior attachment (8%). The attachment also has been noted to have a distinct bifurcate origin in rare instances.[10]

The biceps tendon is widest at its origin and progressively narrows. Habermeyer and associates[8] reported the tendon to be 8.2 × 2.8 mm wide at its origin and 9.2 cm

FIGURE 5

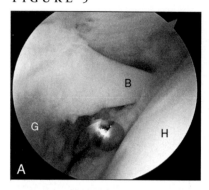 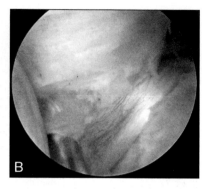 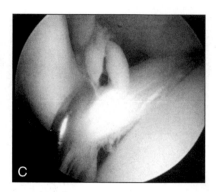

Arthroscopic images of the right shoulder with the patient in the beach chair position. A complete diagnostic arthroscopy includes visualization of the entire intra-articular biceps tendon (B). **A,** An initial inspection reveals some fibrillation at the anterior aspect of the tendon just distal to its origin from the superior glenoid rim (G). **B,** When a probe is used to pull the bicipital groove portion of the tendon into the joint, synovitis is noted. **C,** The bicipital groove portion of the tendon should be routinely inspected because severe degenerative lesions of the biceps necessitating tenodesis or tenotomy occasionally are discovered. H = humeral head.

long. The tendon traverses obliquely over the humeral head and exits the glenohumeral joint beneath the transverse humeral ligament. It is encased in a synovial sheath that ends in a blind pouch at the distal end of the intertubercular sulcus, or bicipital groove. The long head of the biceps tendon is, therefore, an intra-articular but extrasynovial structure.

Initial investigation of the tendon and labrum should identify the type of origin and qualify any synovitis or degenerative fibrillation of tissue. A probe inserted through the anterior portal can be used to lift and attempt to displace the superior labral origin. Pathologic conditions also have been reported to occur in the portion of the biceps tendon that resides in the bicipital groove (Figure 5). To examine this hidden segment of tendon, a probe or shaver is used to provide inferior traction, thereby pulling a few centimeters of tendon into the joint.

ROTATOR INTERVAL

Situated between the anterior border of the supraspinatus and the superior edge of the subscapularis, the rotator interval extends medially to the base of the coracoid and laterally to the transverse humeral ligament. The coracohumeral ligament (CHL), superior glenohumeral ligament (SGHL), joint capsule, biceps tendon, and the superior aspect of the middle glenohumeral ligament (MGHL) all lie within the rotator interval. The CHL

originates on the dorsolateral aspect of the proximal third of the coracoid process; however, the origin of the SGHL is less consistent. The rotator interval has been reported to be the primary restraint to inferior glenohumeral translation and external rotation with the arm adducted.[11-13]

In a recent report, Jost and associates[12] described the rotator interval in great detail. Cadaveric dissection revealed two medial layers and, where the interval tissue crosses the articular surface margin on the humeral head, four lateral layers. Medially, the rotator interval comprises the CHL superficially and the SGHL and joint capsule in the deeper layer. The CHL and the SGHL form the roof and the floor, respectively, of a sling that functions as the primary restraint to biceps subluxation from the intertubercular groove (Figure 6). Laterally, the most superficial layer is composed of superficial fibers of the CHL that blend into the insertions of the supraspinatus and subscapularis. The second layer consists of crisscrossing fibers of the supraspinatus and subscapularis that blend into each other and portions of the CHL. Deep fibers of the CHL form the third layer, the main portion of which inserts on the greater tuberosity with relatively fewer fibers extending to the lesser tuberosity and forming the roof of the biceps sling. The fourth or bottom layer is composed of the SGHL and joint capsule. The SGHL inserts at the fovea capitis of the head of the humerus, adjacent to the superior margin of the lesser tuberosity, and forms the floor of the biceps sling.

FIGURE 6

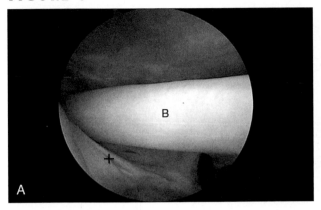
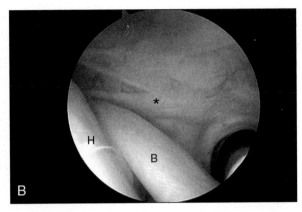

Arthroscopic images of the left shoulder with the patient in the beach chair position. **A,** The superior glenohumeral ligament (+) forms the floor of the biceps sling that functions to help prevent medial displacement of the biceps tendon (B). **B,** When the biceps is drawn into the joint, deep fibers of the coracohumeral ligament (asterisk) are seen to form the roof of this stabilizing sling. H = humeral head.

FIGURE 7

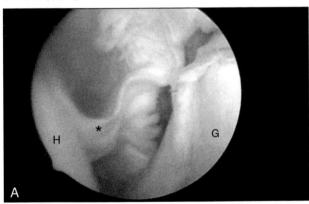
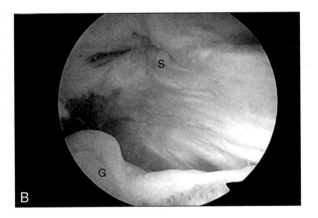

Arthroscopic views of the left shoulder with the patient in the beach chair position. A biceps tendon rupture accompanies this rotator interval tear and helps to expose a hidden lesion. **A,** Lateral disruption of the rotator interval, including the superior glenohumeral and coracohumeral ligaments, has produced slack in the biceps sling (asterisk). **B,** Tearing of the superior rolled edge of the subscapularis (S) from its lateral insertion may be difficult to visualize and frequently is missed in open surgery for isolated anterior supraspinatus tears. G = glenoid; H = humeral head.

This lateral extent of the rotator interval is critical in providing a force that stabilizes the biceps tendon against medial subluxation. The deep anterior fibers of the CHL, the insertion of the SGHL, and the insertion of the subscapularis tendon become confluent laterally and form a sling for the biceps tendon at its medial entrance to the intertubercular groove. Injuries of the lateral interval and biceps sling have been termed hidden lesions[14] (Figure 7). Shoulder elevation and internal rotation provide optimal arthroscopic visualization of these structures. The presence of a lesion of the lateral rotator interval or superior subscapularis indicates biceps instability and vice versa.

Tetro and associates[15] examined rotator interval anatomy relevant to an arthroscopic release for adhesive capsulitis. The interval was reported to be an average of 22-mm wide at the glenoid rim. This measurement is useful when the superior border of the subscapularis is obscured by scar tissue or is otherwise not readily visible. The anterior border of the biceps tendon was used

FIGURE 8

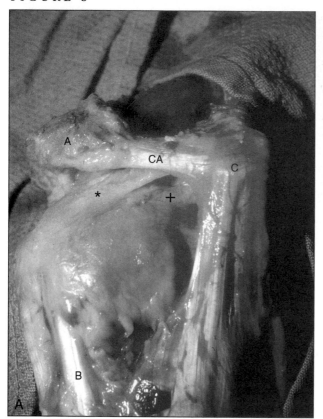

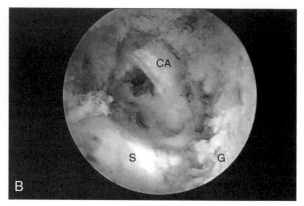

Arthroscopic view of the left shoulder with the patient in the beach chair position. **A,** The coracohumeral (asterisk) and superior glenohumeral ligaments (+) are tensioned when this cadaveric right shoulder is externally rotated in adduction. **B,** The coracoacromial ligament (CA) overlies the medial rotator interval and defines the depth of release in the arthroscopic treatment of adhesive capsulitis. A = acromion; B = biceps tendon; C = coracoid tip; S = subscapularis tendon; G = glenoid. (*Reproduced with permission from Tetro AM, Bauer G, Hollstien SB, Yamaguchi K: Arthroscopic release of the rotator interval and coracohumeral ligament: An anatomic study in cadavers. Arthroscopy 2002;18:145-150.*)

as a landmark for the superior end point of dissection to prevent injury to the anterior border of the supraspinatus. The coracoacromial ligament (CAL) was reported to overlie the CHL at the level of the glenoid rim and served as a guide to the depth of dissection needed to fully release the CHL (Figure 8). There is a mean of 6.2 mm between the structures; however, if scar tissue has filled this space, as in frozen shoulder, the dissection could be up to 1 cm or more. A complete arthroscopic release of the CHL was reported to be consistently possible if the interval was released from the anterior biceps to the superior subscapularis at the glenoid rim until the fibers of the CAL were observed in the depth of the dissection. When these parameters were used, no inadvertent injury to the surrounding musculature was noted, and the musculocutaneous nerve was found to be a minimum of 2 cm away from the deepest portion of the dissection.[15]

GLENOID LABRUM

The glenoid labrum is a circumferential rim of fibrocartilaginous tissue attached to the margin of the glenoid fossa. Functionally, it increases the concavity of the relatively flat osseous glenoid and serves as a stable attachment site for the biceps origin, glenohumeral ligaments, and capsule. Thus, it is a critical static stabilizer of the shoulder and prone to injury with traumatic or recurrent subluxations and dislocations.

Evaluation of this structure is complicated because numerous normal variants have been recognized. A thorough knowledge of normal labral variability is critical to avoid treatment errors. This variability tends to increase from the inferior labrum, which has a fairly consistent presentation, to the superior labrum, which is highly variable. Thus, a normal labrum can be defined as peripherally continuous with the joint capsule and the periosteum of the scapular neck and centrally

FIGURE 9

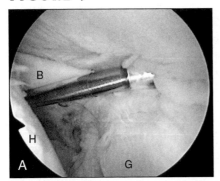 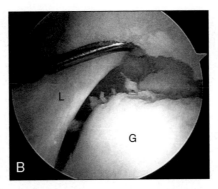 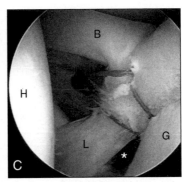

Arthroscopic views of the left shoulder with the patient in the beach chair position. **A,** A mobile biceps origin is displaced medially and found to have a firm medial attachment. Normal hyaline cartilage extends over the superior glenoid rim (G). **B,** A traumatic SLAP lesion as evidenced by the exposed bone on the superior glenoid neck and the lack of medial attachment. **C,** The apparent lesion of the anterosuperior labrum (L) should be recognized as a sublabral foramen (asterisk). This anatomic variant does not display signs of trauma and should not be incorporated into the SLAP repair to avoid unnecessary restriction of external rotation. B = intra-articular biceps tendon; H = humeral head.

attached to the hyaline cartilage of the glenoid through a narrow fibrocartilaginous transition zone. This definition will be used as a basis for comparison of variants. Cooper and associates[16] reported significant differences between the inferior and superior aspects of the labrum. The labrum above the glenoid equator was noted to be triangular or meniscoid in shape, often draping over the articular margin and frequently having a mobile attachment. In contrast, the labrum below the glenoid equator was consistently seen as a rounded extension of the articular surface and usually was attached firmly to the articular surface and the inferior glenohumeral ligament (IGHL).

The superior glenoid is the only location on the glenoid rim where hyaline cartilage has been reported to extend over the rim and project 3 to 4 mm medially.[16,17] Occasionally, a mobile biceps-labral complex can be appreciated. In this instance, the complex is attached medial to the rim and can be mistaken for a superior labral anterior and posterior (SLAP) lesion, as described by Snyder and associates.[18] Determining whether a mobile superior glenoid labrum is a normal variant or pathologic can be difficult. The key to distinguishing the normal variant from a true SLAP lesion is to recognize both the presence of normal hyaline articular cartilage extending over the superior rim of the glenoid and a smooth transition to the labral undersurface (Figure 9).

Davidson and Rivenburgh[17] also have attempted to characterize the normal mobile superior labrum. In 191

consecutive shoulder arthroscopies, 49 shoulders (26%) had articular cartilage on the supraglenoid tubercle, a mobile labrum, and no evidence of superior labral injury. The authors also identified three types of superior labral shapes: triangular (44%), meniscoid (38%), and bumper-shaped (18%). The type of superior labrum had no correlation to a mobile labrum or SLAP tear found at the time of arthroscopy. True superior labral pathology is recognized by the absence of articular cartilage under a highly mobile or dynamically unstable biceps-labral complex with evidence of tissue injury. Parentis and associates[19] described a test for evaluating unstable superior labral lesions in which the fully distended joint is suctioned, causing an unstable superior labrum to pull away from the glenoid rim.

SLAP lesions frequently are associated with pathology elsewhere in the shoulder. Kim and associates[20] noted that 88% (123 of 139) of SLAP lesions in their series were associated with other intra-articular abnormalities. In particular, SLAP lesions frequently were seen with partial-thickness supraspinatus tears, Bankart lesions, and glenohumeral arthritis. Their report highlights the need for a thorough diagnostic arthroscopy, and the expectation that multiple pathologic lesions will be found, especially in the injured shoulder.

Although not considered a classic, posttraumatic SLAP lesion, a "peel-back" mechanism of labral injury has been described by Burkart and Morgan.[21] Repetitive torsional forces, such as those seen during the late cock-

FIGURE 10

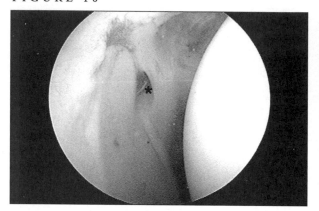

Arthroscopic view of the right shoulder with the patient in the beach chair position. Normal anterosuperior sublabral foramen (asterisk).

FIGURE 11

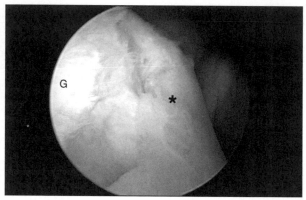

Arthroscopic view of the left shoulder with the patient in the lateral decubitus position viewed from the anterosuperior portal looking inferiorly along the anterior glenoid rim (G). An avulsion of the anteroinferior labrum and anterior band of the inferior glenohumeral ligament (asterisk) from the glenoid rim is noted. This Bankart lesion has displaced medially and healed to the medial glenoid neck.

ing phase of throwing, are believed to peel back the biceps origin and posterosuperior labrum from the glenoid rim, resulting in a posteriorly based type II SLAP lesion. This lesion is demonstrated during arthroscopy by placing the arm in extreme abduction and external rotation, which displaces the posterosuperior labral tear. Dynamic assessment of the labral attachment is necessary when fraying or degeneration of the posterosuperior labrum is seen, particularly in throwing athletes who present with subtle instability and a positive relocation test.

Studies of the anterosuperior labrum have revealed three primary anatomic variations. In a recent study of 546 patients who underwent shoulder arthroscopy, Rao and associates[22] identified 18 patients (3.3%) with a sublabral foramen, defined as a sulcus, between a well-developed anterosuperior labrum and the glenoid rim (Figure 10). Forty-seven (8.6%) patients had a sublabral foramen with a cord-like MGHL, whereas 8 (1.5%) had a completely absent anterosuperior labrum and a cord-like MGHL arising from the superior labrum at the biceps origin, the so-called Buford complex. Williams and associates,[23] in their original description, also reported the Buford complex with an incidence of 1.5% (3 of 200). Ilahi and associates[24] recently noted a slightly higher incidence of sublabral foramen (18.5%) and Buford complex (6.5%) in a consecutive series of 108 shoulder arthroscopies. If a Buford complex is mistaken for a labral avulsion and reattached to the neck of the glenoid, a severely painful restriction of external rota-

tion and elevation is likely to result. Anterior labral deficiency superior to the midglenoid notch rarely reflects true pathology.

Any tissue fraying or labral detachment below the glenoid equator should be considered pathologic. Because both the anterior and posterior portions of the inferior labrum are more consistent in their appearance and relationship to surrounding structures, the identification of pathology is more straightforward. The inferior labrum can be visualized from a posterior viewing portal in most shoulders. Damage to the humeral articular cartilage must be minimized while performing a complete diagnostic arthroscopy. In tight shoulders when visualization of the anteroinferior labrum is difficult, the arthroscope should be driven over the humeral articular surface toward the rotator interval before dropping the tip inferiorly. This procedure takes advantage of the smooth cannula as a head retractor and minimizes cutting of the articular surface with the edges of the camera tip. The posteroinferior labrum usually can be visualized from a posterior portal as well unless the shoulder is tight, when an anterior viewing portal and the drive-through technique should be used. The posterosuperior labrum must be viewed from anterior if pathology is suspected.

The inferior labrum typically is attached firmly to the cartilage centrally and to the capsuloligamentous com-

FIGURE 12

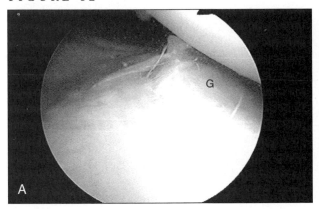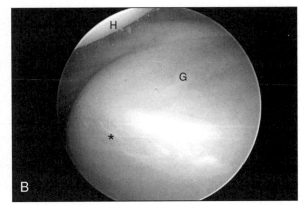

Arthroscopic views of the left shoulder with the patient in the lateral decubitus position. **A,** A posteroinferior labral avulsion from the glenoid rim (G) is visualized from the posterior portal in a patient with recurrent posterior instability. **B,** A marginal crack (asterisk) of the posteroinferior labrum, as described by Kim and associates,[5,26] is seen in this patient with multidirectional instability and should be probed to investigate for the presence of a concealed avulsion. Note the capacious joint space in this shoulder with a positive drive-through sign.

plex laterally. It appears as a thick, rounded extension of the cartilage surface. The anterior band of the IGHL is intimately attached to both the glenoid and the labrum at the 4 o'clock position. The Bankart lesion can be identified by an avulsion of the capsulolabral complex from the anteroinferior glenoid rim. Identification of an acute lesion is fairly straightforward; however, when the lesion is encountered late, it can be less obvious. The anterior ligamentous periosteal sleeve avulsion lesion can be seen in the latter situation, when the IGHL-labrum complex has been avulsed and then healed in a medially displaced position along the anteroinferior glenoid neck[25] (Figure 11).

There is a gradual transition back to a more loosely attached labrum posteriorly from inferior to superior. Cooper and associates[16] noted that the posteroinferior labrum and the capsule in this region, which represents the posterior band of the IGHL, are slightly thinner. Kim and associates[5,26-28] reported extensively on lesions of the posteroinferior labrum in patients with posterior instability. Any marginal posteroinferior labral cracks must be investigated thoroughly with a probe because labral avulsions can appear normal on superficial inspection.[29] Loss of chondrolabral height also has been reported in patients with recurrent posteroinferior instability, although a cause-effect relationship has not been clarified.[27] The significance of anterior and posterior separation of the labrum from the articular margin

probably is similar (Figure 12).

Internal impingement, first described by Walch, is a condition in which the articular surface of the rotator cuff makes contact with the posterosuperior glenoid and labrum during shoulder abduction, external rotation, and extension.[30-33] When this normal contact becomes a pathologic kissing lesion is not fully understood, but it seems to be related to fatigue in overhead throwing athletes. Partial-thickness articular-sided tears of the supra- and infraspinatus and degeneration of the posterosuperior labrum are the arthroscopic hallmarks of this process. Posterosuperior labral detachment, lesions of the long head of the biceps, and chondromalacia or fissuring of the posterosuperior glenoid articular cartilage also can be identified.

GLENOHUMERAL LIGAMENTS

The SGHL, MGHL, and IGHL play a crucial role in static glenohumeral stability, depending on the position of the humerus. When viewed externally, the glenohumeral capsule is featureless. When the internal surface is examined arthroscopically, however, the deep capsule has discrete thickenings. Strain measurement and selective cutting studies have shown that the glenohumeral ligaments provide specific functional contributions to glenohumeral stability.[13,29,34-36] The significant normal variation in these ligaments must be recognized so that appropriate treatment strategies can be formulated.

FIGURE 13

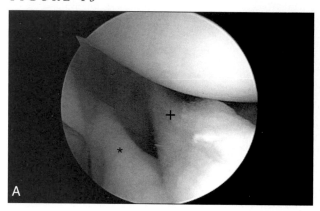
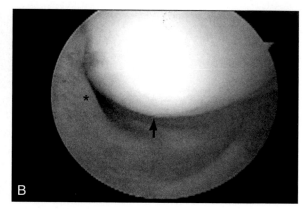

Arthroscopic views of the right shoulder with the patient in the lateral decubitus position. **A,** The MGHL (asterisk) and anterior band of the IGHL (+) as seen from the anterosuperior portal of a right shoulder. **B,** The posterior band of the IGHL (asterisk) and intervening axillary pouch (*arrowhead*) as seen in beach chair orientation from the posterior viewing portal.

They typically can be viewed from the posterior portal, although their most lateral insertions onto the humerus may require a 70° arthroscope or an anterior viewing portal.

The SGHL originates from the supraglenoid tubercle, anterior to the biceps origin, and inserts at the humeral fovea capitis, adjacent to the superior margin of the lesser tuberosity just medial to the bicipital tuberosity. The SGHL often is obscured by the biceps tendon, however, and may not be discretely recognizable. In approximately 17% of specimens, it originates solely from the glenoid labrum at approximately the 1 o'clock position on a right shoulder, sharing a common origin with the MGHL.[37] The presence of the SGHL is consistent, but its thickness is quite variable. It usually is found superior to the long head of the biceps and may be obscured by the biceps as the ligament courses laterally. In addition, the SGHL can be difficult to identify if it is thin and rudimentary; it is visualized best with the arm in adduction and external rotation. The function of the SGHL has not been delineated clearly from that of the CHL, but together they form a restraining sling to the long head of the biceps tendon and limit inferior translation and external rotation when the arm is adducted.

The MGHL arises from the supraglenoid tubercle and anterosuperior glenoid labrum immediately below the origin of the SGHL. The superomedial aspect of the ligament is contained within the rotator interval, and its insertion blends with portions of the subscapularis ten-

don 2 cm medial to that tendon's insertion on the lesser tuberosity.[36] Arthroscopically, the MGHL is best visualized in its midportion, where it obliquely crosses the upper rolled tendon edge of the subscapularis. The MGHL is present 85% of the time, averaging 3.6 mm in diameter and 18 mm in length, although its size and shape vary widely.[37] It is not seen as consistently as the SGHL and has the greatest number of normal variants among the three ligaments. The normal MGHL has been described as broad and flat and somewhat confluent with the anterior band of the IGHL. In approximately 9% of the population, the MGHL is cord-like and associated with a sublabral foramen, possibly contributing to the misperception that the labrum is pathologically deficient.[23] It is an important restraint to anterior translation in the midrange of shoulder abduction. The MGHL usually represents the leading edge of a Bankart lesion. Patients with a sublabral foramen and a Bankart lesion should be recognized to avoid repairing a normal cord-like ligament to the anterior glenoid rim and unnecessarily restricting glenohumeral motion.

The IGHL complex consists of an anterior band, a posterior band, and an intervening thickening of the capsule, termed the axial pouch[38] (Figure 13). The anterior band originates between the 2 and 4 o'clock positions, whereas the posterior band originates between the 7 and 9 o'clock positions on the glenoid and labrum or the neck of the glenoid just adjacent to the labrum. Two types of origin have been reported for the anteroinferior capsulolabrum, the location of the anterior band of the IGHL.[39] A type I origin in which the ligament originates from the glenoid rim, labrum, and neck is present 80% of the time. In a type II origin (20%), the ligament originates directly from the glenoid neck, adjacent to the glenoid labrum. In another study of 52 fetal and embryonic shoulders, 77% attached directly to the capsule, and 23% attached medially to the scapular neck with a free-standing labrum, creating an anterior pouch,[40] suggesting that the degree of normal variation in the IGHL origin is congenital rather than acquired.

The ligament inserts onto the anatomic neck of the humerus in one of two configurations, either as a collar just inferior to the articular margin or as a V with the axillary pouch inserting at the apex distal to the articular cartilage.[38] The ligament can be visualized best arthroscopically with the arm in an abducted position. The posterior band becomes prominent with internal rotation, and the anterior band becomes prominent with external rotation. Whether the posterior band of the IGHL represents a discrete ligament or a capsular thickening is disputed. Regardless, there is little dispute that the IGHL complex is the main static constraint to glenohumeral stability with the arm in the abducted position.

The Bankart lesion, described previously, involves injury to the MGHL and the anterior band of the IGHL in addition to the labrum.[41] In patients with recurrent anterior instability, some degree of capsular stretching must occur in addition to or instead of a Bankart lesion.[42] Therefore, simply repairing the Bankart lesion without addressing the capsular and ligamentous laxity will not fully address the pathology and likely will lead to a higher rate of failure. This situation has led to the concept of the arthroscopic capsulolabral repair and involves a capsular plication and superior shift of the IGHL onto the glenoid rim.

Uncommonly, an avulsion of the IGHL from the lateral humeral insertion can result from a traumatic anterior dislocation. This finding has been termed the HAGL lesion (humeral avulsion of glenohumeral ligament) and has been described as occurring in up to 9.3% of patients with anterior instability undergoing arthroscopic evaluation.[43,44] This lesion is best seen either from an anterior portal or with the use of a 70° arthroscope from the traditional posterior portal. It is important to remember the HAGL lesion when an unstable shoulder has an unexpectedly normal-appearing anteroinferior glenoid and labrum.

Finally, there is no single normal pattern of development or insertion of the glenohumeral ligaments. There are variations in the individual size, shape, and insertion of each ligament, as well as collective differences in their pattern. The ligaments are evaluated and classified with respect to their general appearance. In the classic pattern each ligament is distinct, with recesses or synovial reflections between them. Occasionally, shoulders demonstrate a pattern of confluence in which the MGHL and IGHL are confluent as one ligament without an intervening recess. Patients with multidirectional instability often have no specific pathologic finding but are noted to have a largely positive drive-through sign and a capacious axillary recess.

ROTATOR CUFF

The rotator cuff consists of four distinct muscles with tendons that coalesce to form a common continuous insertion on the proximal humerus. The subscapularis forms the anterior cuff, inserting on the lesser tuberosity, whereas the posterior cuff comprises the supraspinatus, infraspinatus, and teres minor, which insert onto the three facets of the greater tuberosity. Functionally, the rotator cuff acts primarily to maintain the midrange stability of the glenohumeral joint during motion. Except for end-range capsular contributions, the rotator cuff is a primary dynamic stabilizer of the shoulder and also provides some power in motion. The rotator cuff remains a significant source of shoulder pain and disability because degenerative changes and tearing increase with age.[45] Thorough understanding of its normal anatomy and tear configuration is essential to recognizing and effectively treating lesions of the rotator cuff.

The subscapularis is a multipennate muscle arising from the subscapularis fossa of the scapula. It is separated from the other muscles of the rotator cuff by the coracoid process and the rotator interval. The superior two thirds has a wide tendinous insertion onto the lesser tuberosity, whereas the inferior third has a narrow direct muscular attachment along the surgical neck. The most superior tendon fibers interdigitate at their insertion with fibers of the supraspinatus because both muscles send fibers to the lesser and greater tuberosities.[46,47] The superior tendinous, or rolled, edge of the subscapularis is easily visible arthroscopically and forms the inferior border of the rotator interval and the arthroscopic triangle. The subscapularis bursa separates the osseous glenoid from the superior tendinous edge of the subscapularis and is lined with synovial membrane. It is best seen through an anterior portal and can be the site of hidden loose bodies. This recess also defines a plane between the superior rolled edge of the subscapularis and the MGHL, IGHL, and capsule and should be developed when anterior capsular release is performed. Medial subluxation of the biceps tendon and/or fraying of the rolled edge of the subscapularis usually represents compromise of the subscapularis insertion and warrants further investigation.

The supraspinatus originates from the supraspinatus fossa of the scapula and passes through the supraspinatus outlet to insert just lateral to the articular margin on the superior facet of the greater tuberosity. The distance from the articular margin to the tendon insertion is less than 1 mm for the anterior 2.1 cm of cuff insertion, after which this distance widens as the posterior cuff inserts lateral to the bare area.[48] The distance between the articular margin and the most medial tendinous insertion is increased for degenerative articular-sided partial-thickness rotator cuff tears. The supraspinatus consists of a significantly larger anterior fusiform muscle belly and a smaller unipennate posterior belly. The anterior belly, however, has an overall thinner tendinous contribution with an average cross-sectional area of 2.6 mm^2 versus 3.1 mm^2 for the posterior belly.[49] Therefore, the larger anterior muscle belly pulls through a smaller tendon area with proportionately greater stress. Priority should be placed on repairing this anterior portion of the tendon during rotator cuff repair because it provides the greatest contractile force.

The infraspinatus is a bipennate muscle that arises from the infraspinatus fossa and is separated into superior and inferior portions by a raphe. Distally, its tendon becomes confluent with tendons of both the supraspinatus and teres minor to form a common insertion on the greater tuberosity. The anterior fibers of the infraspinatus tendon have been found to merge inseparably with the posterior supraspinatus tendon approximately 15 mm from their insertion, making the interval between these two tendons arthroscopically indistinguishable.[47] A similar blending of fibers occurs between the infraspinatus and teres minor, inferiorly. Approximately 29% to 62% of the infraspinatus tendon inserts anterior to the leading edge of the humeral bare area, depending on the method of measurement.[48,50] More-

FIGURE 14

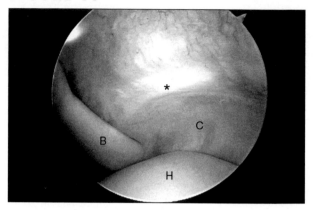

Arthroscopic view of the right shoulder with the patient in the beach chair position. The rotator cable (asterisk) as viewed from the posterior portal. Note the relative avascularity of the rotator crescent (C). B = biceps tendon; H = humeral head.

over, the posterior edge of the infraspinatus inserts a mean of 8.6 to 11.7 mm posterior to the leading edge of the bare area. This has implications for the characterization of full-thickness rotator cuff tears. Tears that extend approximately 1 cm posterior to the leading edge of the bare area involve the entire infraspinatus.

The concept of a posterior rotator interval has been developed with implications for rotator cuff mobilization in retracted posterior cuff tears.[51,52] The posterior rotator interval is defined by the spine of the scapula as the infraspinatus and supraspinatus course laterally and then merge toward their insertion. It averages 49.4 mm in length from the spinoglenoid notch to the confluence of the tendons and is devoid of muscle or tendon.[52] When a massive cuff tear is retracted and scarred posteriorly, dividing the interval between these two muscles and corresponding tendons back toward the spinoglenoid notch may be essential to realigning the tendons for repair or partial repair.

The teres minor is a fusiform muscle that originates from the inferolateral border of the scapula and inserts onto the greater tuberosity at the lateral edge of the bare area, approximately 15 mm from the articular surface. Like the subscapularis, it has both a broad superior tendinous insertion and a narrower inferior muscular attachment onto the surgical neck.

When the articular surface of the rotator cuff is evaluated arthroscopically, a thickened transverse band of tissue is visualized running medial and perpendicular

FIGURE 15

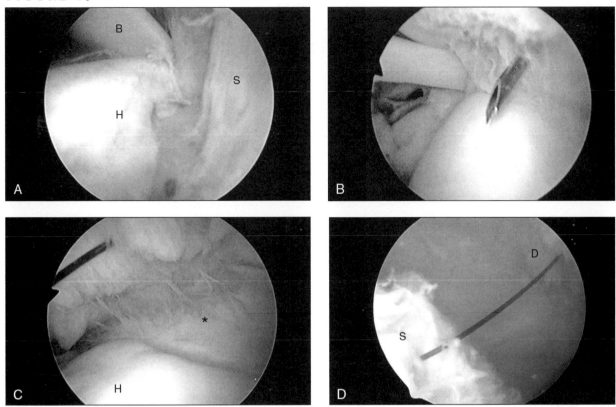

Arthroscopic views through the posterior portal of the right shoulder with the patient in the beach chair position. **A,** The normal supraspinatus tendon (S) can insert up to 1 to 2 mm lateral to the articular margin of the humeral head (H). **B,** A spinal needle is used to pass monofilament suture through the region of a suspected partial-thickness tear. **C,** An articular-sided partial-thickness rotator cuff tear of the supraspinatus is visualized. The medial-lateral dimension of the exposed greater tuberosity (asterisk) can aid in approximating the percentage of tendon that has torn. **D,** The suture is used to identify the bursal surface of the tear during subsequent subacromial arthroscopy. B = biceps tendon; D = subdeltoid fascia.

to the insertion of the cuff. First described by Clark and associates, this transverse band, more commonly known as the rotator cable, is a deep extension of the coracohumeral ligament that traverses posterior from the anterior supraspinatus to the posterior border of the infraspinatus.[47,53,54] The rotator cable defines the medial border of the rotator crescent, that portion of cuff that is tightly adherent to the underlying glenohumeral capsule, where most articular-sided degenerative rotator cuff lesions are reported to occur. The synovial vasculature of the undersurface of the rotator cuff does not appear to continue lateral to the rotator cable because the rotator crescent tissue appears avascular (Figure 14). In a study by Burkhart and associates,[53] the size of the rotator crescent averaged 41 mm in its anterior-poste-

rior dimension and 14 mm in its medial-lateral dimension, while the cable was 12- × 4.7-mm thick. Burkhart[55] hypothesized that the rotator cable acts as a tension line to disperse stress across the rotator cuff insertion and to resist superior head migration when tears are present within the crescent.

Historically, the treatment of partial-thickness tears has been based on the percentage of tendon thickness involved, which can be difficult to measure. The percentage of tendon thickness involved in a partial-thickness tear can be determined more accurately by measuring the distance from the most medial remaining rotator cuff insertion to the articular margin (Figure 15). Dugas and associates[48] provided the foundation for a more scientific estimation of partial-thickness tears

FIGURE 16

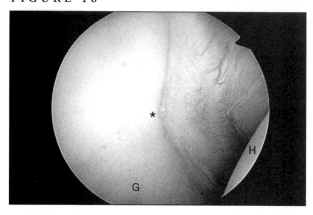

Arthroscopic view of the right shoulder with the patient in the beach chair position. The midglenoid notch (asterisk) of the anterior glenoid rim is an intra-articular landmark of the approximate origin of the anterior band of the IGHL and roughly divides the superior from the inferior glenoid (G). H = humeral head.

in their study of the rotator cuff insertions in 20 cadaveric shoulders. If the dimensions of the tendinous footprint are known, then a percentage estimate of partial-thickness tearing can be made. The mean medial-lateral dimension of the supraspinatus footprint was found to be 12.7 mm; the infraspinatus was slightly wider at 13.4 mm, and the teres minor slightly narrower at 11.4 mm. Therefore, when an articular-sided tear exists, and the distance from the articular margin to the most medial tendon fibers is 7 to 8 mm, approximately 50% of the supraspinatus is involved (when the 1 mm between the articular margin and the normal cuff insertion is included). This finding has been substantiated in another recent report on the dimensions of the supraspinatus footprint.[56] However, this calculation cannot be used if the tear involves the posterior infraspinatus where the tendon inserts several millimeters from the articular margin, lateral to the bare area.

Gerber and associates[57] classified a massive full-thickness rotator cuff tear as a tear that involves two entire tendons rather than using the older, more arbitrary 5-cm measurement. Because the tendon insertions blend seamlessly together, the size of a full-thickness cuff tear is more easily estimated when the anterior-posterior dimension of the cuff insertions is known. The supraspinatus and infraspinatus both have a mean anterior-posterior dimension of approximately 1.6 cm, with the teres minor

having a slightly longer insertion of approximately 2 cm.[48] Minagawa and associates[50] reported slightly longer dimensions and blending of the supraspinatus and infraspinatus insertions. Based on the results of these two studies, a full-thickness rotator cuff tear that extends approximately 3.2 to 3.5 cm posteriorly from the rotator interval would be considered a massive tear according to Gerber's classification. Intra-articular landmarks should be used when attempting to size tears. The posterior edge of the intra-articular biceps tendon or, alternatively, the posterior aspect of the bicipital groove in the setting of a biceps rupture, is used to approximate the anterior edge of the supraspinatus. The posterior edge of the supraspinatus inserts a mean of 4 to 5 mm anterior to the leading edge of the bare area, which is 21 to 26 mm posterior to the bicipital groove, whereas the posterior edge of the infraspinatus inserts approximately 8 to 12 mm posterior to the leading edge of the bare area.[48,50] Therefore, a tear that extends approximately 1 cm posterior to the leading edge of the bare area would be assumed to include the entire infraspinatus.

GLENOHUMERAL SKELETAL ANATOMY

Glenohumeral osteoarticular anatomy is generally consistent from an arthroscopic perspective. Arthroscopic inspection of the anterior glenoid rim reveals an indentation termed the midglenoid notch (Figure 16) that is just superior to the glenoid's equator. This notch emphasizes the glenoid's inverted comma or pear shape. The articular surfaces of the glenoid and humeral head conform nearly perfectly. The radius of curvature of the articular surfaces differs by less than 1% despite their having widely different osseous radii of curvature.[58] An analysis of version has revealed a glenoid twist with an average of 13° of retroversion superiorly decreasing to an average of 3° of retroversion inferiorly.[59] Kim and associates[27] reported that shoulders with atraumatic posteroinferior instability had greater retroversion of both the osseous and the chondrolabral portion of the inferior glenoid, as seen on MR arthrogram, when compared with age-matched normal shoulders.

Because the osseous glenoid is relatively flat, the articular cartilage and labrum function to decrease the radius of curvature. The articular cartilage is relatively thick at the periphery but thins in the center, often resulting in a visible bare spot. The bare spot, which easily can be

FIGURE 17

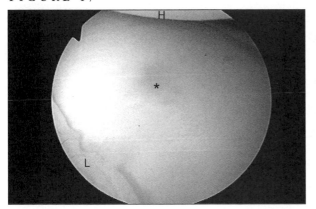

Arthroscopic view through the anterosuperior portal of the right shoulder with the patient in the lateral decubitus position. The glenoid bare spot (asterisk) represents the normal area of thin articular cartilage that lies at the geometric center of the inferior glenoid. It should not be mistaken for chondromalacia. H = humeral head; L = anterior glenoid labrum.

FIGURE 18

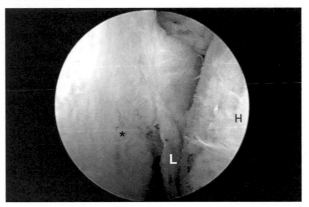

Arthroscopic view of the right shoulder with the patient in the beach chair position. Osteoarthritis in this shoulder is evidenced by the presence of articular cartilage fibrillation and fragmentation on both the glenoid and the humeral head (H). Asterisk = glenoid bare spot; L = anteroinferior glenoid labrum.

mistaken for early osteoarthritis or chondromalacia (Figure 17), has been reported to lie at the geometric center of the inferior glenoid (that area of the glenoid below the midglenoid notch), equidistant from the anterior and posterior rims.[60] This location can be used to aid in the quantification of bone loss in traumatic instability when using an intra-articular ruler, such as that found on some arthroscopic probes. The anteroinferior or posteroinferior bone loss or compression, when significant, can produce what Burkhart and De Beer[61] and Lo and associates[62] have termed the "inverted pear" glenoid.

One recent study evaluated the osseous anatomy of the superior glenoid rim with respect to anchor placement in SLAP repairs.[63] The ideal angle of insertion was determined to be approximately 30° relative to the glenoid face. At this angle optimal bony purchase was obtained between the cortex of the glenoid face and the superior neck. The margin for error decreases slightly, but significantly, in the posterosuperior glenoid rim.

The humeral head articular surface is ovoid and roughly three times the surface area of the glenoid. At any given time, only a quarter to a third of the humeral head articulates with the glenoid. The humeral head articular surface should appear smooth, without evidence of chondromalacia except for the posterolateral aspect of the head (Figure 18). Devoid of cartilage, this

region lateral to the articular surface and medial to the posterior cuff insertion has been termed the bare area; the name is not to be confused with the bare spot of the glenoid (Figure 19). The humeral bare area can appear quite irregular but has a smooth transition with the articular cartilage. It should not be mistaken for a Hill-Sachs lesion, which also is found posteriorly, usually more medial, and has a more irregular transition to articular cartilage. A dynamic assessment can determine if the long axis of the Hill-Sachs lesion engages the anterior glenoid parallel to the rim in the functional position of abduction and external rotation. The presence of an inverted pear glenoid and/or engaging Hill-Sachs lesion has implications for the success of arthroscopic Bankart repairs.[61]

ACROMIAL ANATOMY

Acromial morphology has been classified into three types: type I, a flat acromion; type II, a curved acromion; and type III, a hooked acromion.[64] Perhaps more important than acromial morphology is the presence or absence of subacromial spurs. These spurs generally originate from the anterolateral acromion at the site of the CA ligament insertion and extend anteromedially toward the coracoid. The presence of subacromial spurs increases with age and is associated with an increased

FIGURE 19

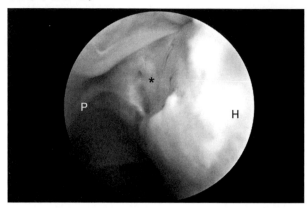

Arthroscopic view through the posterior portal of the left shoulder with the patient in the beach chair position. The humeral bare area (asterisk) is normally seen at the posterior aspect of the humeral head where the rotator cuff inserts lateral to the articular margin. The leading edge of the bare area can be used as an intra-articular landmark to quantify the involvement of the infraspinatus tendon in full-thickness rotator cuff tears as discussed previously. H = humeral head articular cartilage; P = posterior capsule and rotator cuff insertion.

prevalence of rotator cuff disease.[65] However, whether these spurs are the cause or result of rotator cuff disease is uncertain.

The dimensions of the acromion were studied by Nicholson and associates[65] in 420 cadaveric scapulas. The acromion is wider at its base, where it arises from the scapular spine, and then narrows anteriorly. In men, the average length of the acromion was 48.5 mm, the anterior width was 19.5 mm, and the average anterior thickness was 7.7 mm. In women, the acromial length was 40.6 mm, the width was 18.4 mm, and the thickness was 6.7 mm. These measurements should guide the amount of bony resection performed during a subacromial decompression. An average acromial thickness of approximately 7 mm is thinner than commonly perceived. An anterior decompression of only 3 mm results in a significant reduction of native acromial thickness. More aggressive resections can increase the risk of compromising the deltoid origin and/or fracturing the acromion.

NEUROVASCULAR ANATOMY

The neurovascular structures most at risk during shoulder arthroscopy include the axillary and suprascapular nerves and, to a much lesser degree, the musculocutaneous nerve. The axillary nerve is a terminal branch of the posterior cord of the brachial plexus. It arises posterior to the coracoid process and courses along the subscapularis passing inferior to it, 3 to 5 mm medial to the musculotendinous junction.[66] The axillary nerve is then in intimate contact with the inferior shoulder capsule.

The axillary nerve branches into anterior and posterior branches at the anterior margin of the long head of the triceps at approximately 6 o'clock relative to the glenoid face. The anterior branch courses lateral to the posterior branch and medial to the posterior circumflex artery.[2] It serves as the primary innervation to the deltoid and is of primary concern during open or miniopen procedures around the shoulder. However, in arthroscopy, the posterior branch is more vulnerable in its position closest to the inferior glenoid labrum.[2,67] Inferior capsular procedures, in particular thermal capsulorrhaphy, appear to predispose the posterior branch to injury.[68] Because both the superior lateral brachial cutaneous (SLBC) nerve and the nerve to the teres minor arise from the posterior branch, injury can be recognized by sensory loss over the lateral deltoid. This finding may indicate loss of teres minor innervation as well.[2] The SLBC nerve courses around the medial border of the deltoid approximately 9 cm inferior to the posterolateral corner of the acromion, safely distanced from appropriately placed posterior portals.

Traveling with the posterior humeral circumflex artery, the anterior branch of the axillary nerve passes through the quadrangular space bound by the teres minor superiorly, the teres major inferiorly, the long head of the triceps medially, and the surgical neck of the humerus laterally. The nerve then courses anteriorly on the undersurface of the deltoid. The nerve is found an average of 5.5 cm distal to the posterolateral corner of the acromion but can be as close as 3.1 cm.[3] Anteriorly, the nerve is an average of 5 cm distal to the anterolateral corner. In one cadaveric study, the axillary nerve was reported to be closer than 5 cm from the acromion at some point in its course in 20% of specimens.[3]

Uno and associates[69] studied the anatomy of the nerve from an intra-articular perspective. In 12 cadavers, the nerve was approximated to the capsule by loose areolar tissue between the 5 and 7 o'clock positions and translated with shoulder motion. The nerve was in close proximity to the anteroinferior glenoid with the shoulder in neutral or internal rotation and extension. The zone of safety increased between the inferior glenoid rim and the axillary nerve with external rotation, abduction, or perpendicular traction, which tended to displace the nerve anterolaterally.

Arthroscopic axillary nerve anatomy was the subject of a recent study in which direct visualization through an intra-articular window and coronal sectioning were used to describe the course of the nerve around the inferior rim.[67] With the arm in 45° of abduction and 20° of flexion, the nerve was an average of 12.4 mm and a minimum of 11 mm from the glenoid rim at the 6 o'clock position. It was observed to be as close as 1 mm from the inferior glenohumeral ligament.

The suprascapular nerve arises from the superolateral aspect of the upper trunk of the brachial plexus. Traveling with the suprascapular artery, the nerve passes through the suprascapular notch and below the superior transverse scapular ligament as the artery courses over. The suprascapular nerve has been noted to rest as close as 2.3 cm from the superior glenoid rim at the suprascapular notch.[70] It sends motor innervation to the supraspinatus muscle as it traverses the muscle's undersurface, adherent to the supraspinatus fossa. It emerges from the posterior edge of the supraspinatus and tracks sharply around the spine of the scapula at the spinoglenoid notch before terminating in multiple motor branches to the infraspinatus. The suprascapular nerve resides a minimum of 1.4 cm from the posterior glenoid rim at the base of the scapular spine.[70] A spinoglenoid ligament has been discovered in 80% of shoulders and forms a fibro-osseous tunnel through which the suprascapular nerve traverses.[71]

A posterior rotator interval release places the suprascapular nerve at some risk if the release is carried to the base of the scapular spine. Dissection in this region should be performed carefully to minimize bleeding and the risk of iatrogenic injury to the nerve. The suprascapular artery and vein usually are found lateral to the nerve at the spinoglenoid notch. Significant bleeding can signify that dissection is nearing the suprascapular nerve. If electrocautery is used, sharp muscular contractions can signify the location of the nerve. Only short bursts of electrocautery should be used in this region because muscular contraction usually will not occur before thermal injury to the nerve. There is some debate as to whether lateral mobilization of a severely retracted massive rotator cuff tear produces clinically relevant stretch injury to the nerve.[72,73] Conversely, reduction or partial repair of a retracted posterosuperior cuff tear may relieve tension on the suprascapular nerve (JJ Warner, MD, et al, Washington, DC, unpublished data presented at the American Shoulder and Elbow Surgeons open meeting, 2005).

Suprascapular nerve compression by a supraglenoid ganglion cyst in combination with a superior labral lesion has been reported.[74] Most commonly, an unstable posterosuperior SLAP lesion permits the pumping of synovial fluid, in a one-way valve fashion, into the supraglenoid space. If a ganglion cyst forms, the suprascapular nerve can be compressed between the cyst and the bone of the spinoglenoid notch, causing pain, signs of infraspinatus atrophy, and external rotation weakness. The supraspinatus is spared because the compression at the spinoglenoid notch is posterior to the supraspinatus innervation. Treatment by needle aspiration or arthroscopic débridement should be accompanied by repair of the superior labral lesion.

The musculocutaneous nerve is a terminal branch of the lateral spinal cord. Its main trunk has been found to enter the coracobrachialis muscle an average of 5.6 to 6.1 cm from the tip of the coracoid with a minimum distance of 3.5 cm.[75,76] The musculocutaneous nerve often has smaller, more proximal branches that enter the muscle a minimum of 2.1 cm from the coracoid tip; therefore, it is potentially at risk during arthroscopic rotator interval release. Tetro and associates[15] noted that a dissection that averaged 11 mm from the coracoid tip, which should be a safe distance from the musculocutaneous nerve, could be required to completely release a thickened rotator interval. Understanding these relationships is important, especially when the interval tissue is thickened, normal planes of dissection have been obliterated, and an electocautery device is being used that can cause distant thermal damage.

The risk of major arterial bleeding in shoulder arthroscopy is exceedingly small, but any bleeding can obscure visualization and make successful intervention difficult. Bleeding rarely will be an issue with glenohumeral arthroscopy; however, it is common to violate vascular zones in subacromial surgery. The maintenance of hypotensive anesthesia, as permitted, is useful in keeping forceful bleeding to a minimum. An awareness of common vascular zones allows the surgeon to anticipate bleeding and effectively use electrocoagulation to provide rapid hemostasis.

The acromial branch of the deltoid artery supplies the AC joint and frequently is encountered during release

FIGURE 20

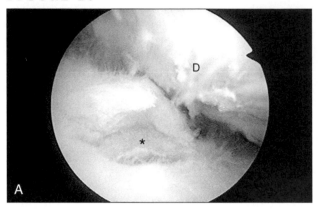
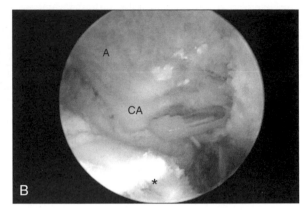

Arthroscopic views of the right shoulder with the patient in the beach chair position. **A,** A bursal-sided partial-thickness supraspinatus tear (asterisk) is visualized in the subacromial space through a posterior viewing portal. **B,** The coracoacromial ligament (CA) is seen to insert along the lateral edge of the acromion (A). D = subdeltoid fascia.

of the CAL at its medial edge. The medial fat zone of the subacromial space is also highly vascular and should be dissected carefully using electrocautery. The supraspinatus artery and vein occasionally can be violated at the base of the scapular spine during posterior interval release. Brisk bleeding in this zone heralds the presence of the supraspinatus nerve, which is found just medial to these vessels.

SUBACROMIAL SPACE

Surgery in the subacromial space requires a focused and expeditious approach because soft-tissue swelling quickly accumulates outside the confines of the gleno-humeral capsule. The acromion, the bursal side of the rotator cuff, and the CAL are major features observed within the subacromial space (Figure 20).

The posterior portal must be in a position that allows the proper insertion angle into the subacromial space for instruments to reach the anterior acromion at the proper working angle. Initial insertion of the trochar is aimed anteromedially along the undersurface of the acromion. The goal is to cannulate the subacromial bursa. Beals and associates[77] reported a thorough investigation, using cadavers of elderly people, of the boundaries of the sub-acromial bursa with respect to arthroscopic surgery. The bursa is situated over the supraspinatus and the very anterior portion of the infraspinatus tendon. The anterolateral corner of the acromion is, in fact, centered over the subacromial bursa. The posterior margin of the bursa is at the midpoint of the anteroposterior dimension of the acromion. The bursa extends medially to the AC joint and laterally under the deltoid. The inferior margin of the lateral subdeltoid bursal reflection is in intimate contact with the axillary nerve.

The anatomy of the CAL has been the subject of multiple anatomic studies.[78-80] The ligament arises from the lateral aspect of the coracoid and courses lateral and superior to the anterior edge of the acromion. Its insertion extends posteriorly along the lateral acromion for a distance of 2 cm from the anterolateral corner. Holt and Allibone[79] described the ligament as quadrangular (48%), Y-shaped (42%), or consisting of one broad band (8%). One specimen in their study had three ligamentous bands, with the third band arising from the inferomedial aspect of the coracoid. In another study, this third band was described as occurring in 14.5% of 124 cadavers.[80] The band was found posteromedial, and the authors suggested that failure to release this band could be a cause of failure in arthroscopic subacromial decompression. The CAL is readily detached anteriorly from the acromion without disturbing the fibers of the anterior deltoid. However, its attachment along the lateral acromion is adherent to the deltoid fascia, starting at the raphe between the anterior and middle deltoid.[78] Care must be taken to prevent detachment of deltoid fibers when releasing the ligament in this area.

The fibers of the anterior deltoid originate via direct

tendinous attachment to the osseous acromion anteriorly and are in jeopardy with anterior subacromial decompression. In one study it was proposed that resection of 4 to 6 mm of anterior acromion would release 41% to 69%, respectively, of the anterior deltoid attachment.[81] One patient with complete deltoid detachment during anterior arthroscopic subacromial decompression has been reported.[82]

REFERENCES

1. Neviaser TJ: Arthroscopy of the shoulder. *Orthop Clin North Am* 1987;18:361-372.

2. Ball CM, Steger T, Galatz LM, Yamaguchi K: The posterior branch of the axillary nerve: An anatomic study. *J Bone Joint Surg Am* 2003;85:1497-1501.

3. Burkhead WZ Jr, Scheinberg RR, Box G: Surgical anatomy of the axillary nerve. *J Shoulder Elbow Surg* 1992;1:31-36.

4. Lo IK, Lind CC, Burkhart SS: Glenohumeral arthroscopy portals established using an outside-in technique: Neurovascular anatomy at risk. *Arthroscopy* 2004;20:596-602.

5. Kim SH, Ha KI, Park JH, et al: Arthroscopic posterior labral repair and capsular shift for traumatic unidirectional recurrent posterior subluxation of the shoulder. *J Bone Joint Surg Am* 2003;85:1479-1487.

6. Davidson PA, Tibone JE: Anterior-inferior (5 o'clock) portal for shoulder arthroscopy. *Arthroscopy* 1995;11: 519-525.

7. Pearsall AW, Holovacs TF, Speer KP: The low anterior five-o'clock portal during arthroscopic shoulder surgery performed in the beach-chair position. *Am J Sports Med* 1999;27:571-574.

8. Habermeyer P, Kaiser E, Knappe M, Kreusser T, Wiedemann E: Functional anatomy and biomechanics of the long biceps tendon. *Unfallchirurg* 1987;90:319-329.

9. Vangsness CT Jr, Jorgenson SS, Watson T, Johnson DL: The origin of the long head of the biceps from the scapula and glenoid labrum: An anatomical study of 100 shoulders. *J Bone Joint Surg Br* 1994;76:951-954.

10. Enad JG: Bifurcate origin of the long head of the biceps tendon. *Arthroscopy* 2004;20:1081-1083.

11. Harryman DT II, Sidles JA, Harris SL, Matsen FA III: The role of the rotator interval capsule in passive motion and stability of the shoulder. *J Bone Joint Surg Am* 1992;74:53-66.

12. Jost B, Koch PP, Gerber C: Anatomy and functional aspects of the rotator interval. *J Shoulder Elbow Surg* 2000;9:336-341.

13. Warner JJ, Deng XH, Warren RF, Torzilli PA: Static capsuloligamentous restraints to superior-inferior translation of the glenohumeral joint. *Am J Sports Med* 1992;20:675-685.

14. Walch G, Nove-Josserand L, Levigne C, Renaud E: Tears of the supraspinatus tendon associated with hidden lesions of the rotator interval. *J Shoulder Elbow Surg* 1994;3:353-360.

15. Tetro AM, Bauer G, Hollstien SB, Yamaguchi K: Arthroscopic release of the rotator interval and coracohumeral ligament: An anatomic study in cadavers. *Arthroscopy* 2002;18:145-150.

16. Cooper DE, Arnoczky SP, O'Brien SJ, Warren RF, DiCarlo E, Allen AA: Anatomy, histology, and vascularity of the glenoid labrum: An anatomical study. *J Bone Joint Surg Am* 1992;74:46-52.

17. Davidson PA, Rivenburgh DW: Mobile superior glenoid labrum: A normal variant or pathologic condition? *Am J Sports Med* 2004;32:962-966.

18. Snyder SJ, Karzel RP, Del Pizzo W, Ferkel RD, Friedman MJ: SLAP lesions of the shoulder. *Arthroscopy* 1990;6: 274-279.

19. Parentis MA, Mohr KJ, ElAttrache NS: Disorders of the superior labrum: Review and treatment guidelines. *Clin Orthop Relat Res* 2002;400:77-87.

20. Kim TK, Queale WS, Cosgarea AJ, McFarland EG: Clinical features of the different types of SLAP lesions: An analysis of one hundred and thirty-nine cases. Superior labrum anterior posterior. *J Bone Joint Surg Am* 2003; 85:66-71.

21. Burkhart SS, Morgan CD: The peel-back mechanism: Its role in producing and extending posterior type II SLAP lesions and its effect on SLAP repair rehabilitation. *Arthroscopy* 1998;14:637-640.

22. Rao AG, Kim TK, Chronopoulos E, McFarland EG: Anatomical variants in the anterosuperior aspect of the glenoid labrum: A statistical analysis of seventy-three cases. *J Bone Joint Surg Am* 2003;85:653-659.

23. Williams MM, Snyder SJ, Buford D Jr: The Buford complex: The "cord-like" middle glenohumeral ligament and absent anterosuperior labrum complex. A normal anatomic capsulolabral variant. *Arthroscopy* 1994;10:241-247.

24. Ilahi OA, Labbe MR, Cosculluela P: Variants of the anterosuperior glenoid labrum and associated pathology. *Arthroscopy* 2002;18:882-886.

25. Neviaser TJ: The anterior labroligamentous periosteal sleeve avulsion lesion: A cause of anterior instability of the shoulder. *Arthroscopy* 1993;9:17-21.

26. Kim SH, Ha KI, Yoo JC, Noh KC: Kim's lesion: An incomplete and concealed avulsion of the posteroinferior labrum in posterior or multidirectional posteroin-

ferior instability of the shoulder. *Arthroscopy* 2004;20:712-720.

27. Kim SH, Noh KC, Park JS, Ryu BD, Oh I: Loss of chondrolabral containment of the glenohumeral joint in atraumatic posteroinferior multidirectional instability. *J Bone Joint Surg Am* 2005;87:92-98.

28. Kim SH, Park JC, Park JS, Oh I: Painful jerk test: A predictor of success in nonoperative treatment of posteroinferior instability of the shoulder. *Am J Sports Med* 2004;32:1849-1855.

29. O'Connell PW, Nuber GW, Mileski RA, Lautenschlager E: The contribution of the glenohumeral ligaments to anterior stability of the shoulder joint. *Am J Sports Med* 1990;18:579-584.

30. Davidson PA, ElAttrache NS, Jobe CM, Jobe FW: Rotator cuff and posterior-superior glenoid labrum injury associated with increased glenohumeral motion: A new site of impingement. *J Shoulder Elbow Surg* 1995;4:384-390.

31. Jobe CM: Superior glenoid impingement: Current concepts. *Clin Orthop Relat Res* 1996;330:98-107.

32. Paley KJ, Jobe FW, Pink MM, Kvitne RS, ElAttrache NS: Arthroscopic findings in the overhand throwing athlete: Evidence for posterior internal impingement of the rotator cuff. *Arthroscopy* 2000;16:35-40.

33. Walch G, Liotard JP, Boileau P, Noel E: Postero-superior glenoid impingement: Another shoulder impingement. *Rev Chir Orthop Reparatrice Appar Mot* 1991;77: 571-574.

34. Debski RE, Wong EK, Woo SL, Sakane M, Fu FH, Warner JJ: In situ force distribution in the glenohumeral joint capsule during anterior-posterior loading. *J Orthop Res* 1999;17:769-776.

35. O'Brien SJ, Schwartz RS, Warren RF, Torzilli PA: Capsular restraints to anterior-posterior motion of the abducted shoulder: A biomechanical study. *J Shoulder Elbow Surg* 1995;4:298-308.

36. Turkel SJ, Panio MW, Marshall JL, Girgis FG: Stabilizing mechanisms preventing anterior dislocation of the glenohumeral joint. *J Bone Joint Surg Am* 1981;63:1208-1217.

37. Steinbeck J, Liljenqvist U, Jerosch J: The anatomy of the glenohumeral ligamentous complex and its contribution to anterior shoulder stability. *J Shoulder Elbow Surg* 1998;7:122-126.

38. O'Brien SJ, Neves MC, Arnoczky SP, et al: The anatomy and histology of the inferior glenohumeral ligament complex of the shoulder. *Am J Sports Med* 1990;18:449-456.

39. Eberly VC, McMahon PJ, Lee TQ: Variation in the glenoid origin of the anteroinferior glenohumeral capsulolabrum. *Clin Orthop Relat Res* 2002;400:26-31.

40. Uhthoff HK, Piscopo M: Anterior capsular redundancy of the shoulder: Congenital or traumatic. An embryological study. *J Bone Joint Surg Br* 1985;67:363-366.

41. Bigliani LU, Pollock RG, Soslowsky LJ, Flatow EL, Pawluk RJ, Mow VC: Tensile properties of the inferior glenohumeral ligament. *J Orthop Res* 1992;10:187-197.

42. Speer KP, Deng X, Borrero S, Torzilli PA, Altchek DA, Warren RF: Biomechanical evaluation of a simulated Bankart lesion. *J Bone Joint Surg Am* 1994;76:1819-1826.

43. Bokor DJ, Conboy VB, Olson C: Anterior instability of the glenohumeral joint with humeral avulsion of the glenohumeral ligament: A review of 41 cases. *J Bone Joint Surg Br* 1999;81:93-96.

44. Wolf EM, Cheng JC, Dickson K: Humeral avulsion of glenohumeral ligaments as a cause of anterior shoulder instability. *Arthroscopy* 1995;11:600-607.

45. Yamaguchi K, Tetro AM, Blam O, Evanoff BA, Teefey SA, Middleton WD: Natural history of asymptomatic rotator cuff tears: A longitudinal analysis of asymptomatic tears detected sonographically. *J Shoulder Elbow Surg* 2001;10:199-203.

46. Boon JM, de Beer MA, Botha D, Maritz NG, Fouche AA: The anatomy of the subscapularis tendon insertion as applied to rotator cuff repair. *J Shoulder Elbow Surg* 2004;13:165-169.

47. Clark JM, Harryman DT II: Tendons, ligaments, and capsule of the rotator cuff: Gross and microscopic anatomy. *J Bone Joint Surg Am* 1992;74:713-725.

48. Dugas JR, Campbell DA, Warren RF, Robie BH, Millett PJ: Anatomy and dimensions of rotator cuff insertions. *J Shoulder Elbow Surg* 2002;11:498-503.

49. Roh MS, Wang VM, April EW, Pollock RG, Bigliani LU, Flatow EL: Anterior and posterior musculotendinous anatomy of the supraspinatus. *J Shoulder Elbow Surg* 2000;9:436-440.

50. Minagawa H, Itoi E, Konno N, et al: Humeral attachment of the supraspinatus and infraspinatus tendons: An anatomic study. *Arthroscopy* 1998;14:302-306.

51. Lo IK, Burkhart SS: Arthroscopic repair of massive, contracted, immobile rotator cuff tears using single and double interval slides: Technique and preliminary results. *Arthroscopy* 2004;20:22-33.

52. Miller SL, Gladstone JN, Cleeman E, Klein MJ, Chiang AS, Flatow EL: Anatomy of the posterior rotator interval: Implications for cuff mobilization. *Clin Orthop Relat Res* 2003;408:152-156.

53. Burkhart SS, Esch JC, Jolson RS: The rotator crescent and rotator cable: An anatomic description of the shoulder's "suspension bridge". *Arthroscopy* 1993;9:611-616.

54. Clark J, Sidles JA, Matsen FA: The relationship of the glenohumeral joint capsule to the rotator cuff. *Clin Orthop Relat Res* 1990;254:29-34.

55. Burkhart SS: Fluoroscopic comparison of kinematic patterns in massive rotator cuff tears: A suspension bridge model. *Clin Orthop Relat Res* 1992;284:144-152.

56. Ruotolo C, Fow JE, Nottage WM: The supraspinatus footprint: An anatomic study of the supraspinatus insertion. *Arthroscopy* 2004;20:246-249.

57. Gerber C, Fuchs B, Hodler J: The results of repair of massive tears of the rotator cuff. *J Bone Joint Surg Am* 2000;82:505-515.

58. Soslowsky LJ, Flatow EL, Bigliani LU, Mow VC: Articular geometry of the glenohumeral joint. *Clin Orthop Relat Res* 1992;285:181-190.

59. Schlemmer B, Dosch JC, Gicquel P, et al: Computed tomographic analysis of humeral retrotorsion and glenoid retroversion. *Rev Chir Orthop Reparatrice Appar Mot* 2002;88:553-560.

60. Burkhart SS, Debeer JF, Tehrany AM, Parten PM: Quantifying glenoid bone loss arthroscopically in shoulder instability. *Arthroscopy* 2002;18:488-491.

61. Burkhart SS, De Beer JF: Traumatic glenohumeral bone defects and their relationship to failure of arthroscopic Bankart repairs: Significance of the inverted-pear glenoid and the humeral engaging Hill-Sachs lesion. *Arthroscopy* 2000;16:677-694.

62. Lo IK, Parten PM, Burkhart SS: The inverted pear glenoid: An indicator of significant glenoid bone loss. *Arthroscopy* 2004;20:169-174.

63. Lehtinen JT, Tingart MJ, Apreleva M, Ticker JB, Warner JJ: Anatomy of the superior glenoid rim: Repair of superior labral anterior to posterior tears. *Am J Sports Med* 2003;31:257-260.

64. Bigliani LU, Morrison DS, April EW: The morphology of the acromion and its relationship to rotator cuff tears. *Orthop Trans* 1986;10:216.

65. Nicholson GP, Goodman DA, Flatow EL, Bigliani LU: The acromion: Morphologic condition and age-related changes. A study of 420 scapulas. *J Shoulder Elbow Surg* 1996;5:1-11.

66. Loomer R, Graham B: Anatomy of the axillary nerve and its relation to inferior capsular shift. *Clin Orthop Relat Res* 1989;243:100-105.

67. Price MR, Tillett ED, Acland RD, Nettleton GS: Determining the relationship of the axillary nerve to the shoulder joint capsule from an arthroscopic perspective. *J Bone Joint Surg Am* 2004;86:2135-2142.

68. Wong KL, Williams GR: Complications of thermal capsulorrhaphy of the shoulder. *J Bone Joint Surg Am* 2001;83(suppl 2):151-155.

69. Uno A, Bain GI, Mehta JA: Arthroscopic relationship of the axillary nerve to the shoulder joint capsule: An anatomic study. *J Shoulder Elbow Surg* 1999;8:226-230.

70. Shishido H, Kikuchi S: Injury of the suprascapular nerve in shoulder surgery: An anatomic study. *J Shoulder Elbow Surg* 2001;10:372-376.

71. Cummins CA, Anderson K, Bowen M, Nuber G, Roth SI: Anatomy and histological characteristics of the spinoglenoid ligament. *J Bone Joint Surg Am* 1998;80:1622-1625.

72. Warner JP, Krushell RJ, Masquelet A, Gerber C: Anatomy and relationships of the suprascapular nerve: Anatomical constraints to mobilization of the supraspinatus and infraspinatus muscles in the management of massive rotator-cuff tears. *J Bone Joint Surg Am* 1992;74:36-45.

73. Zanotti RM, Carpenter JE, Blasier RB, Greenfield ML, Adler RS, Bromberg MB: The low incidence of suprascapular nerve injury after primary repair of massive rotator cuff tears. *J Shoulder Elbow Surg* 1997;6:258-264.

74. Piatt BE, Hawkins RJ, Fritz RC, Ho CP, Wolf E, Schickendantz M: Clinical evaluation and treatment of spinoglenoid notch ganglion cysts. *J Shoulder Elbow Surg* 2002;11:600-604.

75. Flatow EL, Bigliani LU, April EW: An anatomic study of the musculocutaneous nerve and its relationship to the coracoid process. *Clin Orthop Relat Res* 1989;244:166-171.

76. Klepps SJ, Goldfarb C, Flatow E, Galatz LM, Yamaguchi K: Anatomic evaluation of the subcoracoid pectoralis major transfer in human cadavers. *J Shoulder Elbow Surg* 2001;10:453-459.

77. Beals TC, Harryman DT II, Lazarus MD: Useful boundaries of the subacromial bursa. *Arthroscopy* 1998;14:465-470.

78. Edelson JG, Luchs J: Aspects of coracoacromial ligament anatomy of interest to the arthroscopic surgeon. *Arthroscopy* 1995;11:715-719.

79. Holt EM, Allibone RO: Anatomic variants of the coracoacromial ligament. *J Shoulder Elbow Surg* 1995;4:370-375.

80. Pieper HG, Radas CB, Krahl H, Blank M: Anatomic variation of the coracoacromial ligament: A macroscopic and microscopic cadaveric study. *J Shoulder Elbow Surg* 1997;6:291-296.

81. Torpey BM, Ikeda K, Weng M, van der Heeden D, Chao EY, McFarland EG: The deltoid muscle origin: Histologic characteristics and effects of subacromial decompression. *Am J Sports Med* 1998;26:379-383.

82. Bonsell S: Detached deltoid during arthroscopic subacromial decompression. *Arthroscopy* 2000;16:745-748.

CHAPTER 2

SUBACROMIAL DECOMPRESSION AND ROTATOR CUFF REPAIR

THEODORE A. BLAINE, MD
SETH MILLER, MD

Recent advances in shoulder arthroscopy have emphasized minimally invasive techniques for subacromial decompression and rotator cuff repair, including arthroscopic and mini-open approaches. In this chapter we review many of the new techniques that have been used to manage rotator cuff disease. However, rotator cuff disease is not a new problem; the first surgical procedure to repair the injured rotator cuff tendon was described by Codman in 1911.[1,2] Open techniques of rotator cuff repair perfected by McLaughlin and Neer have been used successfully for the past 5 decades.[3-8] The goal of arthroscopic treatment of rotator cuff disease, therefore, is to follow the same principles of surgical treatment using smaller incisions with less trauma to the patient. Although new treatments will continue to emerge as the understanding of rotator cuff disease advances, the surgical goals continue to include decompression of the subacromial space and a tension-free repair of the tendon to allow healing of the bone.

PATHOPHYSIOLOGY

Despite the advances in both diagnosis and surgical treatment of rotator cuff disorders, the exact etiology of rotator cuff tendinopathy is not fully understood. Both intrinsic and extrinsic theories of tendon injury have been proposed. In 1921, Meyer[9] proposed an extratendinous theory in which tendon and capsular tears were believed to be secondary to frictional contact of the greater tuberosity on the acromion. This theory was contrary to that proposed by Lindblom[10] in 1939, in which injury was thought to be secondary to tension in the fascicles of the tendon aponeurosis. Codman[1] later emphasized the contribution of trauma to tendon injury. Finally, Neer[5] turned the focus of etiology back to the acromion when he described impingement syndrome in 1972.

Recent investigations also addressed the role of the subacromial bursa in rotator cuff pathology. Although some believe that the subacromial bursa contributes to the healing process leading to the repair of a degenerated rotator cuff tendon, others believe that it contributes to the pain and degeneration of the tendons.[11-16] Increased inflammatory mediators and afferent nerve endings and their products recently have been identified in inflamed subacromial bursa.[17-22] Our recent investigations have also demonstrated that these inflammatory mediators may be reduced directly by cyclooxygenase inhibitors and steroids.[23,24] These findings support the importance of the subacromial bursa in rotator cuff disease and suggest a mechanism of action for many medications that reduce inflammation in the subacromial bursa.

Currently, the etiology of rotator cuff tendinopathy is believed to be multifactorial, and the relative contributions of the etiologic factors remain to be determined. Rotator cuff tears are common, and their incidence increases with advancing age. Trauma can be associated in up to 58% of patients, and the incidence is particularly high in overhead throwing athletes (30%) and laborers (23%). Nonsurgical treatment is successful in most patients, although results are highly variable and depend on several factors, including patient age, tear size, and level of function.[24-30] Surgical principles of rotator cuff repair are much the same as those proposed by McLaughlin[3] in 1944: reestablish the continuity of the cuff mechanism, obtain a tension-free repair, and create a smooth acromial surface to limit extrinsic impingement. Although the role of acromioplasty recently has been questioned, we believe that a limited acromioplasty of the anteroinferior acromion, which does not compromise the deltoid origin, is an important component of surgical treatment.[31-39] In most series, the results of arthroscopic treatment are comparable to those of open techniques, with less patient morbidity, and, in experienced hands, less time in surgery.

CLINICAL EVALUATION

History and Physical Examination

Pain is the most common symptom in patients with rotator cuff disease. Although acute rotator cuff tears can be caused by sudden trauma, especially in the presence of shoulder dislocation, the pain of rotator cuff disease often occurs insidiously and usually cannot be related to a specific inciting event. The pain often radiates down the arm but does not localize below the elbow. The pain radiation is attributed to the subacromial and subdeltoid bursae, which are rich in nerve endings and extend down to the deltoid insertion on the arm. The pain usually is aggravated by overhead activities, but rest pain and night pain also may be present. Additional symptoms, including weakness and inability to raise the arm, often indicate a larger tear.

Physical examination should include visual inspection to identify any deltoid or spinatus muscle atrophy. A bulge in the proximal arm may indicate rupture of the biceps tendon, whereas the presence of a "fluid sign" (a large effusion in the anterosuperior shoulder) may indicate a massive rotator cuff tear consistent with rotator cuff tear arthropathy. Ecchymosis may be present in an acute injury. Palpation will reveal tenderness over the greater tuberosity.

Both passive and active range of motion should be assessed. Although passive range of motion usually is preserved with rotator cuff tears, mild stiffness from posterior capsular tightness can exacerbate impingement symptoms, and, although rare, a secondary adhesive capsulitis may occur in some patients. In patients with severe impingement, an arc of pain will be present with passive motion. Provocative tests should be performed, including both the Neer test and Hawkins impingement sign. In the classic Neer impingement test, passive forward elevation of the arm in the scapular plane produces pain, which is then eliminated by injection of 10 mL of lidocaine into the subacromial space. The Hawkins impingement sign is present when internal rotation of an arm that is abducted to 90° produces pain in the subacromial space. Biceps and labral pathology are also important to consider. The Yergason's and Speed's tests can elicit symptoms of biceps tears, whereas the active compression test is useful in diagnosing superior labral tears.

Although strength may be normal in some patients with small full-thickness rotator cuff tears, weakness is usually present with larger tears. Pain occasionally complicates the clinical examination, and a subacromial lidocaine injection may be useful to distinguish pain from true weakness. Strength in forward elevation and external rotation should be closely examined. Patients with large tears have a positive lag or drop sign, indicating weakness of external rotation. A positive drop sign, which is the inability to maintain neutral rotation with the arm at the side, usually indicates a tear of the infraspinatus and teres minor. Patients with massive tears often cannot actively elevate the arm above 90°. Patients with weakness that is not painful require an expanded differential diagnosis. Neurologic lesions, including cervical radiculopathy, brachial neuritis, suprascapular neuropathy, or syringomyelia, must be considered.

Specific attention should be paid to potential tears of the subscapularis tendon, which often are undiagnosed. These tears are more common in the presence of acute trauma and anterior shoulder dislocation, although they also may occur in chronic massive rotator cuff tears. The lift-off test is performed by internally rotating the arm behind the back and asking the patient to keep the hand away from the small of the back. An inability to do so suggests subscapularis insufficiency. An easier test to perform in the presence of significant pain or stiffness is the belly-press test in which the patient is asked to maintain the elbow in a forward position with the hand pressed on the belly. Inability to do so or side-to-side weakness on this examination also may indicate a subscapularis tear.

Imaging Studies

Routine radiographic evaluation should include supraspinatus outlet, axillary, and AP radiographs in neutral, internal, and external rotation. Further imaging may be necessary in the patient who has not responded to nonsurgical treatment. Arthrography, ultrasonography, and MRI can confirm the presence or absence of a rotator cuff tear. Ultrasonography is advantageous because it is noninvasive and inexpensive; however, it is usually useful only for identifying full-thickness rotator cuff tears. MRI is the preferred modality because it more clearly provides information regarding tear size, tear location, and tissue quality. MRI should be obtained in the scapular plane to evaluate the infraspinatus attachment and to obtain more proximal cuts to assess muscle atrophy. Atrophy of the spinatus muscles may predict the inability to completely repair the rotator cuff. Axillary images are needed to evaluate the subscapularis tendon and subluxation, dislocation, or rupture of the long head of the biceps.

INDICATIONS

Nonsurgical Treatment

Nonsurgical treatment of rotator cuff tears and impingement syndrome is successful in 33% to 92% of patients.[29,40-42] Treatment consists of rest and avoidance of provocative activities. A trial of nonsteroidal anti-inflammatory drugs should be attempted if not contraindicated by other patient factors. Physical therapy can be helpful in maintaining motion, increasing rotator cuff strength, and decreasing inflammation and pain. Passive range-of-motion exercises should be combined with resistive exercises with the arm below the horizontal. Therapeutic modalities, such as heat, ultrasound, iontophoresis, and phonophoresis also can be of value.

If these nonsurgical treatment modalities are unsuccessful, subacromial injection of steroid medication should be considered. Injection may be performed from the anterior, lateral, or posterior approach. Usually no more than three injections should be given before the patient is counseled to have surgical treatment.

Surgical Treatment

When a rotator cuff tear is identified in combination with pain or functional deficit that is not responsive to nonsurgical treatment, surgery is indicated. Nonsurgical treatment typically is continued for 3 to 6 months before surgery is contemplated. More urgent surgery may be necessary in young patients with acute tears and in older patients who have acute extensions of chronic tears. The ability to repair the rotator cuff may be improved in these patients when surgery is performed within the first 3 weeks after injury.

With the advent of arthroscopic techniques that pose less morbidity to the patient, some have advocated lowering the threshold to surgical treatment. However, arthroscopic treatment will not change the biology of tendon healing; therefore, the same length of time is required for postoperative protection and physical therapy to ensure tendon healing. In fact, with arthroscopic treatment, patients often need to be advised to progress slowly in postoperative physical therapy because they may have less pain from the surgery.

TECHNIQUES

General Principles

We routinely perform arthroscopic rotator cuff repair as an outpatient procedure with the patient in the beach chair position under regional anesthesia (interscalene block). Hypotensive (systolic blood pressure < 100 mm Hg) anesthesia facilitates the procedure. The bed is turned 45°. Once the patient is carefully positioned, standard diagnostic arthroscopy is performed. We prefer gravity inflow with epinephrine in the first three bags only. The arm is supported with a hydraulic arm holder so that it can be positioned freely in space during the procedure (Figure 1).

Portal Placement

Accurate portal placement is a critical feature of shoulder arthroscopy (Figure 2). Guidelines for portal placement follow; however, subtle variation in anatomy and patient morphology can impact portal placement. A standard posteroinferior portal, approximately 2 cm inferior and 1 to 2 cm medial to the posterolateral corner of the acromion, is the starting portal. This portal is modified to coincide with the palpable soft spot. The posterolateral portal is made 1 cm off of the posterolateral corner of the acromion, and the lateral portal is aligned with the posterior aspect of the AC joint. The anterior portal is made just lateral to the coracoid process and is the portal used for intra-articular surgery performed through the rotator interval. If AC joint

FIGURE 1

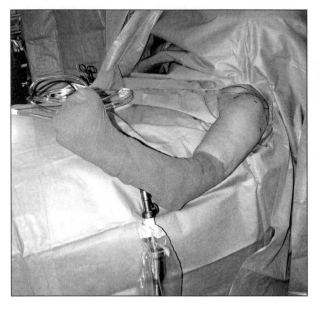

A hydraulic arm positioner is used to position the arm freely in space.

FIGURE 2

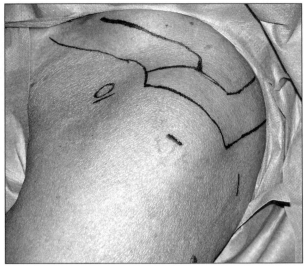

The right shoulder is prepared and draped with the patient in the beach chair position. The commonly used portals (posterior, midlateral, and anterior) are shown.

resection is planned, this portal is moved slightly superiorly. Clear cannulas are used in each of the portals so that visualization is not compromised by the cannulas themselves. We routinely place cannulas in each of the portals as soon as a rotator cuff tear is identified and repair is elected. This placement allows us to move efficiently from portal to portal and to both visualize and instrument the tear from all angles.

Diagnostic Arthroscopy

Arthroscopic examination of the glenohumeral joint is a critical component of arthroscopic treatment of rotator cuff disease. Any intra-articular pathology is addressed appropriately, and the rotator cuff is then carefully examined and probed. The insertion and excursion of the subscapularis tendon is examined and repaired as needed. The insertion and integrity of the footprints of the supraspinatus and infraspinatus are also probed; a monofilament stitch can be placed to demarcate a partial articular-sided tear.

Subacromial Decompression

Once the intra-articular surgery, which may include repair of the subscapularis, is complete, attention is

turned to the subacromial space, and a complete bursectomy is performed, including a complete bursectomy of the lateral gutter. Bursectomy is an important component of the procedure, both to allow appropriate visualization of the tendon and also to remove inflammatory mediators present in the bursa.[23,24] The rotator cuff is inspected through the posterior and midlateral portals to assess the extent of the tear.

Anterior acromioplasty usually is performed after the repair of a rotator cuff tear, unless the acromial morphology prevents satisfactory placement of an anterior cannula. The amount of bone removed varies depending on the preoperative acromial morphology, but removal of only a few millimeters of the anterior acromion usually is required (Figure 3, *A*). Great care should be taken to protect the deltoid origin during this procedure. When bone removal is performed from the inside out, the periosteum of the acromion and the adjacent deltoid origin can be visualized as a white line of tissue attached to the anterior acromion (Figure 3, *B*). Preservation of this tissue ensures preservation of the deltoid origin. Acromioplasty is not performed in all patients. In a patient with a massive irreparable rotator cuff tear, the coracoacromial arch is preserved to prevent humeral head migration superior to the coracoacromial arch.

FIGURE 3

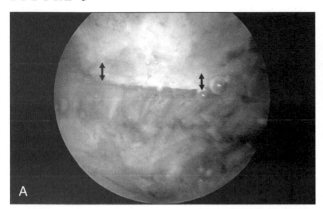 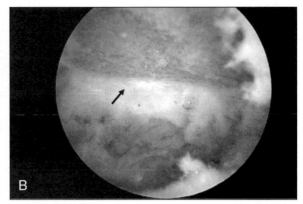

A, Arthroscopic view from the posterior portal of the right shoulder showing a subacromial spur from the anteroinferior acromion. Arrows indicate amount of bone removed. **B,** The same view after acromioplasty. The arrow points to the white line of the periosteum/deltoid fascia.

FIGURE 4

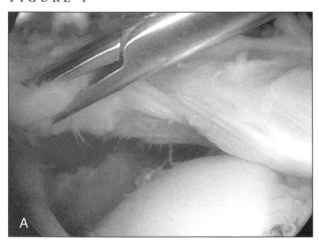 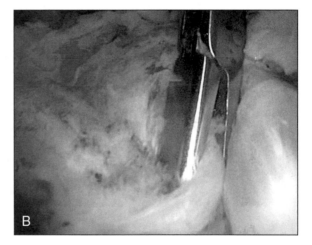

Arthroscopic views from the lateral portal of the right shoulder. A grasper is used to estimate the ability of the tear to be closed with side-to-side sutures (margin convergence technique).

SURGICAL PROCEDURE

Complete Tears

After viewing and understanding the morphology and pattern of tear reduction, a soft-tissue grasper is placed sequentially through both cannulas to determine if the tear reduces with a straight lateral, anterolateral, or posterolateral reduction. As the reduction is performed, the apex of the tear often will be identified (when present), dictating whether a side-to-side suture is needed (Figure 4). In some shoulders, a traction suture may be placed to assist in tear reduction. A variety of suture-passing instruments are available that allow sutures to be passed in a single step (Figure 5). The greater tuberosity is then denuded of fibrous tissue and excoriated to bleeding bone, although a bony trough is not made because cortical bone is needed for anchor purchase (Figure 6).

If required, side-to-side sutures (margin convergence technique) are passed first (Figure 7). This step may be completed with a suture passer or with tissue penetrators passed percutaneously or through cannulas. In some

FIGURE 5

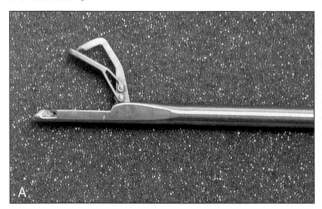
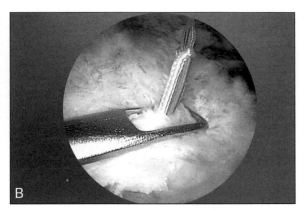

A, Photograph of a viper suture passing instrument (Arthrex, Naples, FL) used in rotator cuff repair. **B,** Arthroscopic view from the lateral portal of the right shoulder showing a scorpion suture passer (Arthrex, Naples, FL) being used to pass sutures through the supraspinatus tendon.

FIGURE 6

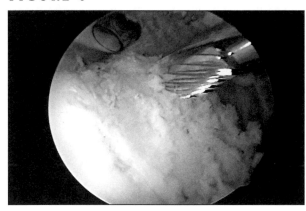

Arthroscopic view from the posterior portal of the right shoulder. A burr is used to débride and abrade the greater tuberosity to stimulate a healing response.

patients, the side-to-side sutures are tied only after remaining sutures and anchors are placed. After tying two or three side-to-side sutures, the ability to pass sutures and place anchors in the tuberosity may be limited; therefore, the surgeon should avoid closing off the working space. Tensioning the side-to-side sutures may help to plan the rest of the repair; these sutures can then be tied before fixing the rotator cuff to the tuberosity. The sutures can be shuttled outside of the anterior or posterior cannula to facilitate the rest of the repair.

A spinal needle is then placed percutaneously along the anterolateral edge of the acromion. The needle is visualized as it approaches the tuberosity, indicating the appropriate direction in which to sequentially insert the suture anchor punch, tap, and anchor, which are placed percutaneously via a small stab incision. An alternative technique involves rotating the arm so that the point of anchor insertion lies directly beneath the lateral cannula, allowing placement through the cannula (Figure 8).

The anchors are placed at a 60° angle and staggered in a medial-to-lateral fashion to reconstruct a wide footprint, when indicated. Double-loaded suture anchors typically are used. Anchor placement requires thorough planning before the first anchor is placed, particularly when double-row fixation is planned. We routinely place the anchor, pass the sutures, and then shuttle the sutures anteriorly, outside of the cannula. The sutures are passed from the portal (anterior, midlateral, or posterior) that facilitates the best tendon purchase and reduction. The arm can be rotated as work is carried out more posteriorly or anteriorly, depending on the tear pattern and mode of fixation. Commercial arm-holding devices are helpful in aligning the tear with portals as needed. The sutures may be passed with a suture passer or with a variety of tissue penetrators passed percutaneously or through cannulas.

Once all of the anchors are placed and sutures are passed, any side-to-side sutures are tied. The sutures placed through anchors are then tied, starting posteriorly and working anteriorly. Meticulous suture management is required, and the anchors should be visualized as the suture limbs are shuttled out to avoid unloading

FIGURE 7

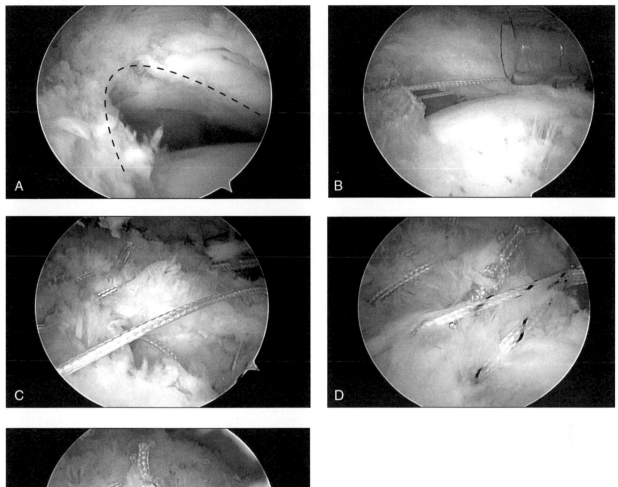

Arthroscopic view from the posterior portal of the right shoulder. **A,** Note the large U-shaped rotator cuff tear (margins indicated by dashed line). **B,** A suture (solid color) has been passed through the anterior and posterior edges of the tear to bring the margins together but has not yet been tied. **C,** The first suture (solid) from the suture anchor placed in the tuberosity is used to close the remaining lateral defect. **D,** The second suture (striped) from the suture anchor is used to complete the repair. **E,** The sutures have all been tied and cut to complete the rotator cuff repair.

the anchors. The sutures should be tied from a cannula that permits the most direct route for tying. We routinely use a sliding knot with three alternating half hitches, alternating the post.

Only the suture limbs that are actively being tied should be in the working cannula. A knot that does not slide easily should not be forced because that can cause the suture to cut out of the soft tissue. Alternating half hitches may be tied instead. The suture limb that passes through the rotator cuff is the post, and the knot is routinely placed on top of the rotator cuff. Once the repair is completed, the rotator cuff should be reduced to the

FIGURE 8

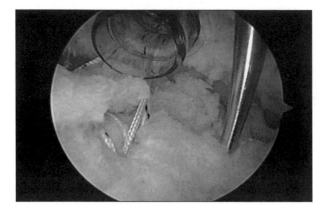

Arthroscopic view from the posterior portal of the right shoulder. Medial row anchors have already been placed. An awl is used to create the path for the lateral row of suture anchors.

footprint at the tuberosity, and secure fixation should be verified as the patient's arm is put through a range of motion. Inadequate fixation should not be accepted, and if additional fixation cannot be achieved through the arthroscope, conversion to a mini-open or open incision may be required.

Massive Tears

Repair of massive rotator cuff tears uses the same techniques and principles required for the repair of smaller tears, including a thorough bursectomy, a three-dimensional understanding of the tear morphology, appropriate capsular and rotator interval releases, an understanding of the direction of reduction, judicious application of various suture passing techniques, and double-row fixation.

After the bursectomy is completed, the standard portals (posterior, posterolateral, midlateral, and anterolateral) are established. Cannulas are placed in the midlateral and anterolateral portals, and the arthroscope in the posterolateral portal. Flexibility and versatility in the working and viewing portals is critical. To repair the tissue, the surgeon needs to adequately see and understand what is being seen. We find it particularly helpful to view the tear from multiple portals and simultaneously use a soft-tissue grasper to reduce the tears from multiple trajectories (portals) (Figure 4). In doing so, the type of tear (ie, elliptical, L-shaped, or reverse L-shaped) often becomes more clear and helps with establishing a plan for repair and position of convergence sutures.

Once the tear pattern is understood, a margin convergence repair is often used in massive tears.[43-48] This repair principle distributes force to the anterior and posterior tear flaps and reduces the overall tension required on the lateral stitches placed at the greater tuberosity. Without margin convergence, inappropriate tensioning and affixing tissue to the lateral aspect of the greater tuberosity is likely to result in failure because the overtensioned tissue is placed at significant biomechanical disadvantage.

If the tear readily reduces, then side-to-side sutures are placed and tied to advance the tissue toward the tuberosity. If the tissue is not compliant, tissue releases are performed. The interval between the rotator cuff and the glenoid is carefully released with an arthroscopic elevator. Superiorly, the coracohumeral ligament may be contracted and safely released. In addition, the rotator cuff may have adhesions between the acromion and deltoid, especially in the revision setting. Radiofrequency devices may be more useful than periosteal elevators because bleeding frequently is encountered in this medial dissection. Awareness of associated neurologic structures is critical, and dissection more than 2 cm medially, especially posteromedially, should be avoided.

If the tissue tension is still too great for repair, an anterior interval slide is performed. The slide can be performed intra- or extra-articularly; we find this differentiation less relevant in a massive retracted tear because the tissue is often at the level of the glenoid. A radiofrequency device or tissue biter is used to longitudinally resect the thickened tissue in the rotator interval along the course of the biceps tendon toward, but not medial to, the coracoid. The anterior slide allows the supraspinatus to be advanced toward the tuberosity. Side-to-side sutures may be passed from interval tissue to the supraspinatus, closing the rotator interval and, more importantly, advancing the supraspinatus. After satisfactory advancement, attention is turned to placing suture anchors.

For massive tears, we prefer a double row of fixation unless the patient has a small surface area of tuberosity or very osteoporotic bone.[49-54] A small surface area in a small patient prohibits the number and placement of suture anchors. Patients with osteoporotic bone often require larger suture anchors (6.5-mm anchor); if the tuberosity does not accommodate two rows of anchors, then a staggered medial-to-lateral (W) configuration is used.

After satisfactory abrasion of the tuberosity, mobilization of the rotator cuff with releases as needed, and the completion of side-to-side sutures, suture anchors are placed through a percutaneous incision off the anterolateral acromion (Figure 9). The medial anchor is placed first, bordering on the edge of the articular surface; the eyelet is aligned parallel to the edge of the tear in contrast to lateral row, or single-row fixation, in which the eyelet is placed perpendicular to the edge of the tear. There are many options for double-row fixation. We recommend placement of a medial row with a single-threaded mattress suture. The medial anchor is placed on the edge of the articular surface, and the mattress suture is placed through the tendon, with careful attention to avoid placing the limbs too close together. The lateral anchor is then placed, and both limbs of the lateral suture are placed through the rotator cuff tissue using simple sutures (Figure 10). One of these sutures is often medial to the medial mattress to create a Mason-Allen configuration or cruciate footprint repair. Once the repair is completed, the sutures are shuttled anteriorly out of the cannula. The same procedure is performed for the middle row, and once again the sutures are shuttled out anteriorly. The arm is internally rotated, and the third (most posterior) row of anchors is placed. We often find that this posterior bone is the weakest, requiring a 6.5-mm anchor, and that the tuberosity will not always accommodate two anchors. In this situation, we place one set of limbs in a mattress fashion and the other limb in a simple fashion. Sutures are tied from posterior to anterior, and the lateral limbs are tied before the medial mattress limbs.

Biceps tenodesis is performed when more than 50% of the tendon is significantly frayed or torn. The anterior edge of supraspinatus tendon tears and biceps pathology have similarities in clinical presentations and may not be distinguished on preoperative MRI. When tenodesis is indicated, soft-tissue tenodesis to the rotator cuff or to an anchor in the bicipital groove often is used. In younger patients or high-demand patients, biceps tenodesis into bone with an interference screw either through an arthroscopic or a subpectoral approach is considered.

Partial-Thickness Bursal Tears

Diagnostic arthroscopy is performed through a standard posterior portal. All intra-articular structures are care-

FIGURE 9

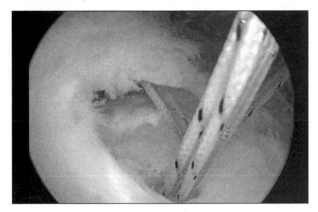

Arthroscopic view from the posterior portal of the right shoulder. A suture anchor has been placed into the greater tuberosity double loaded with sutures. There is a large U-shaped tear of the supraspinatus tendon with exposed greater tuberosity.

fully probed through the rotator interval. Attention is then turned to the subacromial space, and a complete bursectomy is performed using a motorized shaver and/or radiofrequency device. The coracoacromial ligament is inspected for fraying. The rotator cuff is inspected from both the posterior and midlateral or lateral portals and carefully probed. Adherent bursal tissue must be removed from the rotator cuff to properly assess its insertion.

Bursal-sided tears are carefully evaluated. Some tears consist of large flaps of rotator cuff tissue, and most of the rotator cuff is significantly frayed and thinned. Partial-thickness tears that are nearly complete are completed and then repaired as described previously. Other partial bursal-sided tears have significant tendon attachment remaining. For these tears, the frayed edges of the bursal-sided flap are identified and gently débrided until normal rotator cuff attachment is visualized anteriorly and posteriorly. The surgeon must be careful not to take down the intact articular fibers of the rotator cuff insertion. The greater tuberosity is abraded to bleeding bone using a round burr. A spinal needle is used to determine the position and angle of approach before an anchor is placed in the tuberosity through a percutaneous stab wound just off the lateral edge of the acromion. A suture lasso can then be used from either the anterior portal or percutaneously to shuttle the suture limbs from the anchor through the full thickness of the rotator cuff—

FIGURE 10

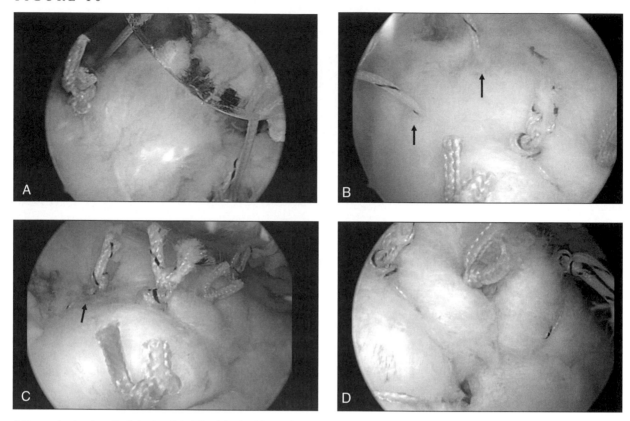

Arthroscopic view from the lateral portal of the right shoulder. **A,** One of the lateral sutures (solid) of the double-row rotator cuff repair has been tied to achieve repair. **B,** The lateral sutures have been tied and cut. A striped suture from the medial anchor row has been passed through the tendon but not yet tied (*arrows*). **C,** The lateral sutures have been tied and cut. The striped suture from the medial anchor row also has been tied (*arrow*). **D,** The lateral sutures have been tied, and a secure repair is seen.

one anteriorly and one posteriorly. Once the lasso is passed through the full thickness of the rotator cuff, the nitinol wire is shuttled out of a cannula along with the more medial of the suture limbs. The nitinol wire is then pulled back out with the suture limb, passing the suture through the full thickness of the rotator cuff. The same procedure is repeated for the posterior limb of the suture. The Neviaser portal also is an option for percutaneous passage through the cuff with suture lassos.

After both sutures are passed through the rotator cuff, the anterior set of sutures is shuttled out of the anterior portal and tied, followed by the posterior set of sutures. Both sutures are tied securely on the bursal surface of the cuff using a sliding knot with three alternating half hitches, which include alternating the post. This technique allows for secure repair without tear completion.

A standard subacromial decompression is performed in these patients because these tears are often secondary to mechanical impingement.

Partial-Thickness Articular Tears

Codman described partial articular-sided cuff tears as rim rents and, more recently, the term PASTA for partial articular-sided tendon avulsion has been used. Some of these tears represent high-grade lesions that are nearly complete (> than 10-mm footprint exposed), and these can be completed and repaired as discussed previously[55-57] (Figure 11). Tears with an exposed footprint of 7 mm can be repaired with a transtendon technique. After the initial intra-articluar evaluation and bursectomy is completed, the arthroscope is returned to the

FIGURE 11

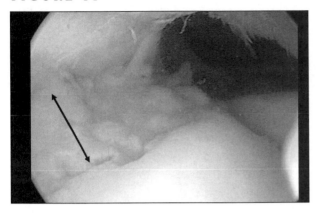

Arthroscopic view from the posterior portal of the left shoulder. More than 7 mm (*arrow*) of exposed supraspinatus footprint is visible, indicating at least a 50% partial-thickness supraspinatus tear.

joint through the posterior portal. The tuberosity is lightly abraded in preparation for repair. A spinal needle is passed through the rotator cuff defect into the exposed tuberosity just lateral to the articular surface. The punch is then passed percutaneously through a small stab incision, followed by the tap and anchor. We typically use a screw-in bioabsorbable suture anchor double-loaded with nonabsorbable sutures. Both limbs of each suture are then brought through the rotator cuff in a retrograde fashion using a sharp suture retrieval device. The limbs of the suture are passed far enough apart to create a bridge of tissue that is brought in contact with the tuberosity when tied. If tendon delamination is noted, the suture can be passed more medially to incorporate this area. If there is enough room on the tuberosity, a second anchor can be placed more posteriorly with sutures passed in a similar manner.

Subscapularis Tears

The overall incidence of subscapularis tears is low compared with that of supraspinatous and infraspinatous tears. Only recently have any publications addressed arthroscopic subscapularis repair.[58-63] The location of these tears can make visualization difficult, particularly if significant swelling has occurred from the arthroscopy. Thus, we believe these tears should be addressed first in patients with multiple tendon tears.

Subscapularis repair requires three portals: anterior, anterolateral, and posterior. Portal sites are localized with

a spinal needle prior to placing cannulas. Partial subscapularis tears involving the superior one third or one half of the tendon are usually less retracted and more readily reduced. Complete tears with retraction can be adherent to the anterior capsule, requiring mobilization. Positioning the arm in flexion and internal rotation improves visualization of the lesser tuberosity footprint. The footprint is prepared with a burr, and the first suture anchor is placed inferiorly into the lesser tuberosity via the anterior portal (Figure 12). One limb of the suture is brought out the anterolateral cannula. A suture lasso is passed from the anterior cannula through the subscapularis tendon at the inferior aspect of the tear. The nitinol loop is used to shuttle the suture limb through the tendon and out the anterior cannula. This technique is repeated for the other suture limb to create a mattress suture. Additional anchors are placed as dictated by the size of the tear. Following completion of the repair, the arm is gently rotated to evaluate the security of the repair and limits for postoperative range of motion. External rotation is usually limited to 40° for 4 to 6 weeks postoperatively.

REHABILITATION

The rehabilitation begins on the first postoperative day, and the program is tailored to the degree of rotator cuff injury and repair. Patients with large or massive tears may be immobilized for 6 weeks, or undergo a modified Neer phase I protocol for 6 weeks that includes pendulum exercises, passive-assist forward elevation to 140°, and passive-assist external rotation (supine) to 30°. Pulley exercises are avoided for the first 6 weeks to protect the rotator cuff repair. Strengthening with isometric exercises is initiated at 6 weeks accompanied by active-assist range of motion. Use of weights is avoided for the first 3 postoperative months to avoid retearing the rotator cuff. Early use of weights has been reported to cause rotator cuff failure. However, resistance exercises with light weights (1 to 3 lb) can be initiated at 12 weeks, progressing to dynamic strengthening exercises at 6 to 8 months. Patients should be aware strength might not be fully restored for 12 to 18 months.

For subacromial decompression only, the rehabilitation program is accelerated. The sling can be removed within the first 1 to 2 weeks, and the patient may use the arm for routine activities of daily living immediately. Return to athletics, particularly overhead sports, how-

FIGURE 12

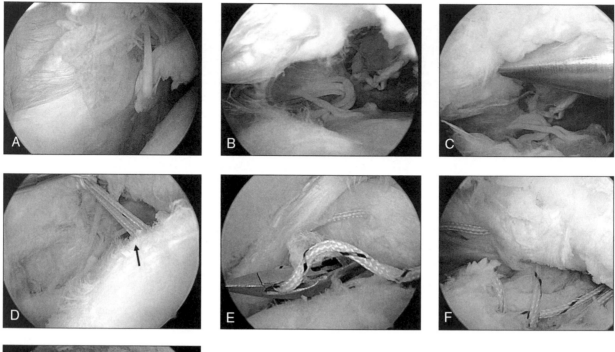

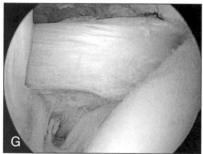

A and B, Arthroscopic views from the posterior portal of the right shoulder demonstrating a complete tear of the subscapularis tendon with detachment from the lesser tuberosity. C, A retractor is pulling the subscapularis off the lesser tuberosity where it has been torn. D, A suture anchor has been placed into the lesser tuberosity, double loaded with two sutures (*arrow*). E, A bird-beak passing instrument (Arthrex, Naples, FL) is used to penetrate the torn subscapularis tendon. The striped suture is grasped and pulled through. The solid suture has already been passed through the tendon. F, The sutures have been passed through the torn subscapularis tendon but not yet tied. G, The torn subscapularis tendon has been repaired to the lesser tuberosity.

ever, should be delayed until 6 to 12 weeks to prevent a postoperative bursitis.

RESULTS

The results of decompression and rotator cuff repair have been evaluated in many series. In general, clinical results, including validated outcome scores and patient satisfaction, have been excellent (90% or better in most series).[43,44,49,64-81] However, results of more recent series, in which tendon integrity was evaluated using ultrasound and MRI, have been less reliable.[69,70,82] In some series, recurrence of rotator cuff tears following arthroscopic repairs has been as high as 90%. These findings

have led to further emphasis on performing the strongest repair possible and repairs that maximize contact of the rotator cuff tendons at their bony insertions. Still, the ability of these technique modifications to enhance tendon healing remains to be seen.

As a result of the benefits achieved by arthroscopic repair (smaller incisions, less deltoid disruption, and patient demand), we continue to favor arthroscopic rotator cuff repair over open repair when tendon repair is indicated. Both single- and double-row repairs are acceptable, although in higher-demand patients with large tears, double-row repair is usually performed. Postoperative rehabilitation must be tailored to the patient;

although a more conservative approach to postoperative physical therapy generally is favored to maximize tendon healing.

The most common complications following decompression and rotator cuff repair include the following: (1) failure to heal, (2) recurrent bursitis, and (3) associated pathology (eg, AC arthrosis). Other less frequent but more severe complications include infection, loose hardware, and deltoid dehiscence with anterosuperior escape. The latter two are the most avoidable. Loose hardware can be prevented by placement of secure anchors; if anchors do not have solid fixation, they should be removed immediately. Anterosuperior escape is a devastating complication that can be avoided by avoiding coracoacromial ligament release and/or acromioplasty in patients with deficient rotator cuff or in repairs of large to massive rotator cuff tears.

REFERENCES

1. Codman E: Complete rupture of the supraspinatus tendon: Operative treatment with report of two successful cases. *Boston Med Surg J* 1911;164:708-710.

2. Codman EA: Rupture of the supraspinatus tendon. 1911. *Clin Orthop Relat Res* 1990;254:3-26.

3. McLaughlin H: Lesions of the musculotendinous cuff of the shoulder: I. The exposure and treatment of tears with retraction. *J Bone Joint Surg Am* 1944;26:31-51.

4. McLaughlin HL: Repair of major cuff ruptures. *Surg Clin North Am* 1963;43:1535-1540.

5. Neer CS II: Anterior acromioplasty for the chronic impingement syndrome in the shoulder: A preliminary report. *J Bone Joint Surg Am* 1972;54:41-50.

6. Neer CS II: Impingement lesions. *Clin Orthop Relat Res* 1983;173:70-77.

7. McLaughlin HL: Lesions of the musculotendinous cuff of the shoulder: The exposure and treatment of tears with retraction. 1944. *Clin Orthop Relat Res* 1994;304:3-9.

8. Neer CS II: Anterior acromioplasty for the chronic impingement syndrome in the shoulder. 1972. *J Bone Joint Surg Am* 2005;87:1399.

9. Meyer A: Further observations on use-destruction in joints. *J Bone Joint Surg* 1922;4:491-511.

10. Lindblom K: On pathogenesis of ruptures of the tendon aponeurosis of the shoulder joint. *Acta Radiol* 1939;20:563-577.

11. Uhthoff HK, Hammond DI, Sarkar K, Hooper GJ, Papoff WJ: The role of the coracoacromial ligament in the impingement syndrome: A clinical, radiological and histological study. *Int Orthop* 1988;12:97-104.

12. Uhthoff HK, Sarkar K: Surgical repair of rotator cuff ruptures: The importance of the subacromial bursa. *J Bone Joint Surg Br* 1991;73:399-401.

13. Uhthoff HK, Sarkar K: Anatomy and pathology of the rotator cuff. *Orthopade* 1995;24:468-474.

14. Uhthoff HK: Recent advances in shoulder surgery. *Curr Opin Rheumatol* 1996;8:154-157.

15. Uhthoff HK, Sano H, Trudel G, Ishii H: Early reactions after reimplantation of the tendon of supraspinatus into bone: A study in rabbits. *J Bone Joint Surg Br* 2000; 82:1072-1076.

16. Uhthoff HK, Trudel G, Himori K: Relevance of pathology and basic research to the surgeon treating rotator cuff disease. *J Orthop Sci* 2003;8:449-456.

17. Gotoh M, Hamada K, Yamakawa H, Tomonaga A, Inoue A, Fukuda H: Significance of granulation tissue in torn supraspinatus insertions: An immunohistochemical study with antibodies against interleukin-1 beta, cathepsin D, and matrix metalloprotease-1. *J Orthop Res* 1997;15:33-39.

18. Gotoh M, Hamada K, Yamakawa H, et al: Increased interleukin-1beta production in the synovium of glenohumeral joints with anterior instability. *J Orthop Res* 1999;17:392-397.

19. Gotoh M, Hamada K, Yamakawa H, et al: Interleukin-1-induced subacromial synovitis and shoulder pain in rotator cuff diseases. *Rheumatology* (Oxford) 2001; 40:995-1001.

20. Santavirta S, Konttinen YT, Antti-Poika I, Nordstrom D: Inflammation of the subacromial bursa in chronic shoulder pain. *Arch Orthop Trauma* Surg 1992;111: 336-340.

21. Soifer TB, Levy HJ, Soifer FM, Kleinbart F, Vigorita V, Bryk E: Neurohistology of the subacromial space. *Arthroscopy* 1996;12:182-186.

22. Ishii H, Brunet JA, Welsh RP, Uhthoff HK: Bursal reactions in rotator cuff tearing, the impingement syndrome, and calcifying tendinitis. *J Shoulder Elbow Surg* 1997;6:131-136.

23. Blaine TA, Kim YS, Voloshin I, et al: The molecular pathophysiology of subacromial bursitis in rotator cuff disease. *J Shoulder Elbow Surg* 2005;14(suppl S)84S-89S.

24. Voloshin I, Gelinas J, Maloney MD, O'Keefe RJ, Bigliani LU, Blaine TA: Proinflammatory cytokines and metalloproteases are expressed in the subacromial bursa in patients with rotator cuff disease. *Arthroscopy* 2005; 21:1076.

25. Hawkins RJ, Kennedy JC: Impingement syndrome in athletes. *Am J Sports Med* 1980;8:151-158.

26. Hawkins RJ, Hobeika PE: Impingement syndrome in the athletic shoulder. *Clin Sports Med* 1983;2:391-405.

27. Bokor DJ, Hawkins RJ, Huckell GH, Angelo RL, Schickendantz MS: Results of nonoperative management of full-thickness tears of the rotator cuff. *Clin Orthop Relat Res* 1993;294:103-110.

28. Hawkins RH, Dunlop R: Nonoperative treatment of rotator cuff tears. *Clin Orthop Relat Res* 1995;321:178-188.

29. Morrison DS, Frogameni AD, Woodworth P: Nonoperative treatment of subacromial impingement syndrome. *J Bone Joint Surg Am* 1997;79:732-737.

30. Wirth MA, Basamania C, Rockwood CA Jr: Nonoperative management of full-thickness tears of the rotator cuff. *Orthop Clin North Am* 1997;28:59-67.

31. Bigliani LU, D'Alessandro DF, Duralde XA, McIlveen SJ: Anterior acromioplasty for subacromial impingement in patients younger than 40 years of age. *Clin Orthop Relat Res* 1989;246:111-116.

32. Bigliani LU, Ticker JB, Flatow EL, Soslowsky LJ, Mow VC: The relationship of acromial architecture to rotator cuff disease. *Clin Sports Med* 1991;10:823-838.

33. Flatow EL, Soslowsky LJ, Ticker JB, et al: Excursion of the rotator cuff under the acromion. Patterns of subacromial contact. *Am J Sports Med* 1994;22:779-788.

34. Bigliani LU, Levine WN: Subacromial impingement syndrome. *J Bone Joint Surg Am* 1997;79:1854-1868.

35. Goldberg BA, Lippitt SB, Matsen FA 3rd: Improvement in comfort and function after cuff repair without acromioplasty. *Clin Orthop Relat Res* 2001;390:142-150.

36. Esch JC, Ozerkis LR, Helgager JA, Kane N, Lilliott N: Arthroscopic subacromial decompression: results according to the degree of rotator cuff tear. *Arthroscopy* 1988;4:241-249.

37. Levy HJ, Gardner RD, Lemak LJ: Arthroscopic subacromial decompression in the treatment of full-thickness rotator cuff tears. *Arthroscopy* 1991;7:8-13.

38. McCallister WV, Parsons IM, Titelman RM, Matsen FA 3rd: Open rotator cuff repair without acromioplasty. *J Bone Joint Surg Am* 2005;87:1278-1283.

39. Zvijac JE, Levy HJ, Lemak LJ: Arthroscopic subacromial decompression in the treatment of full thickness rotator cuff tears: A 3- to 6-year follow-up. *Arthroscopy* 1994;10:518-523.

40. Hawkins RJ, Abrams JS: Impingement syndrome in the absence of rotator cuff tear (stages 1 and 2). *Orthop Clin North Am* 1987;18:373-382.

41. Dalton SE: The conservative management of rotator cuff disorders. *Br J Rheumatol* 1994;33:663-667.

42. Baltaci G: Subacromial impingement syndrome in athletes: prevention and exercise programs. *Acta Orthop Traumatol Turc* 2003;37(suppl 1):128-138.

43. Burkhart SS, Danaceau SM, Pearce CE Jr: Arthroscopic rotator cuff repair: Analysis of results by tear size and by repair technique-margin convergence versus direct tendon-to-bone repair. *Arthroscopy* 2001;17:905-912.

44. Rebuzzi E, Coletti N, Schiavetti S, Giusto F: Arthroscopic rotator cuff repair in patients older than 60 years. *Arthroscopy* 2005;21:48-54.

45. Burkhart SS, Athanasiou KA, Wirth MA: Margin convergence: a method of reducing strain in massive rotator cuff tears. *Arthroscopy* 1996;12:335-338.

46. Burkhart SS: Arthroscopic treatment of massive rotator cuff tears. *Clin Orthop Relat Res* 2001;390:107-118.

47. Burkhart SS: The principle of margin convergence in rotator cuff repair as a means of strain reduction at the tear margin. *Ann Biomed Eng* 2004;32:166-170.

48. Richards DP, Burkhart SS: Margin convergence of the posterior rotator cuff to the biceps tendon. *Arthroscopy* 2004;20:771-775.

49. Mazzocca AD, Millett PJ, Guanche CA, Santangelo SA, Arciero RA: Arthroscopic single-row versus double-row suture anchor rotator cuff repair. *Am J Sports Med* 2005;33:1861-1868.

50. Millett PJ, Mazzocca A, Guanche CA: Mattress double anchor footprint repair: A novel, arthroscopic rotator cuff repair technique. *Arthroscopy* 2004;20:875-879.

51. Ahmad CS, Levine WN, Bigliani LU: Arthroscopic rotator cuff repair. *Orthopedics* 2004;27:570-574.

52. Ahmad CS, Stewart AM, Izquierdo R, Bigliani LU: Tendon-bone interface motion in transosseous suture and suture anchor rotator cuff repair techniques. *Am J Sports Med* 2005;33:1667-1671.

53. Park MC, Cadet ER, Levine WN, Bigliani LU, Ahmad CS: Tendon-to-bone pressure distributions at a repaired rotator cuff footprint using transosseous suture and suture anchor fixation techniques. *Am J Sports Med* 2005;33:1154-1159.

54. Kim DH, Elattrache NS, Tibone JE, et al: Biomechanical comparison of a single-row versus double-row suture anchor technique for rotator cuff repair. *Am J Sports Med* 2006;34:407-414.

55. Miller SL, Hazrati Y, Cornwall R, et al: Failed surgical management of partial thickness rotator cuff tears. *Orthopedics* 2002;25:1255-1257.

56. Gartsman GM, Milne JC: Articular surface partial-thickness rotator cuff tears. *J Shoulder Elbow Surg* 1995;4:409-415.

57. McConville OR, Iannotti JP: Partial-thickness tears of the rotator cuff: Evaluation and management. *J Am Acad Orthop Surg* 1999;7:32-43.

58. Bennett WF: Arthroscopic repair of isolated subscapularis tears: A prospective cohort with 2- to 4-year follow-up. *Arthroscopy* 2003;19:131-143.

59. Travis RD, Burkhead WZ Jr, Doane R: Technique for repair of the subscapularis tendon. *Orthop Clin North Am* 2001;32:495-500.

60. Mansat P, Frankle MA, Cofield RH: Tears in the subscapularis tendon: descriptive analysis and results of surgical repair. *Joint Bone Spine* 2003;70:342-347.

61. Richards DP, Burkhart SS, Lo IK: Subscapularis tears: Arthroscopic repair techniques. *Orthop Clin North Am* 2003;34:485-498.

62. Kreuz PC, Remiger A, Erggelet C, Hinterwimmer S, Niemeyer P, Gachter A: Isolated and combined tears of the subscapularis tendon. *Am J Sports Med* 2005;33: 1831-1837.

63. Lyons RP, Green A: Subscapularis tendon tears. *J Am Acad Orthop Surg* 2005;13:353-363.

64. Blaine TA, Freehill MQ, Bigliani LU: Technique of open rotator cuff repair. *Instr Course Lect* 2001;50:43-52.

65. Murray TF Jr, Lajtai G, Mileski RM, Snyder SJ: Arthroscopic repair of medium to large full-thickness rotator cuff tears: Outcome at 2- to 6-year follow-up. *J Shoulder Elbow Surg* 2002;11:19-24.

66. Bennett WF: Arthroscopic repair of full-thickness supraspinatus tears (small-to-medium): A prospective study with 2- to 4-year follow-up. *Arthroscopy* 2003;19: 249-256.

67. Lo IK, Burkhart SS: Double-row arthroscopic rotator cuff repair: Re-establishing the footprint of the rotator cuff. *Arthroscopy* 2003;19:1035-1042.

68. Boszotta H, Prunner K: Arthroscopically assisted rotator cuff repair. *Arthroscopy* 2004;20:620-626.

69. Galatz LM, Ball CM, Teefey SA, Middleton WD, Yamaguchi K: The outcome and repair integrity of completely arthroscopically repaired large and massive rotator cuff tears. *J Bone Joint Surg Am* 2004;86-A: 219-224.

70. Klepps S, Bishop J, Lin J: Prospective evaluation of the effect of rotator cuff integrity on the outcome of open rotator cuff repairs. *Am J Sports Med* 2004;32:1716-1722.

71. Park JY, Chung KT, Yoo MJ: A serial comparison of arthroscopic repairs for partial- and full-thickness rotator cuff tears. *Arthroscopy* 2004;20:705-711.

72. Buess E, Steuber KU, Waibl B: Open versus arthroscopic rotator cuff repair: A comparative view of 96 cases. *Arthroscopy* 2005;21:597-604.

73. Ide J, Maeda S, Takagi K: A comparison of arthroscopic and open rotator cuff repair. *Arthroscopy* 2005;21:1090-1098.

74. Tauro JC: Arthroscopic rotator cuff repair: Analysis of technique and results at 2- and 3-year follow-up. *Arthroscopy* 1998;14:45-51.

75. Wilson F, Hinov V, Adams G: Arthroscopic repair of full-thickness tears of the rotator cuff: 2- to 14-year follow-up. *Arthroscopy* 2002;18:136-144.

76. Severud EL, Ruotolo C, Abbott DD, Nottage WM: All-arthroscopic versus mini-open rotator cuff repair: A long-term retrospective outcome comparison. *Arthroscopy* 2003;19:234-238.

77. Wolf EM, Pennington WT, Agrawal V: Arthroscopic rotator cuff repair: 4- to 10-year results. *Arthroscopy* 2004;20:5-12.

78. Sauerbrey AM, Getz CL, Piancastelli M, Iannotti JP, Ramsey ML, Williams GR Jr: Arthroscopic versus mini-open rotator cuff repair: A comparison of clinical outcome. *Arthroscopy* 2005;21:1415-1420.

79. Sugaya H, Maeda K, Matsuki K, Moriishi J: Functional and structural outcome after arthroscopic full-thickness rotator cuff repair: Single-row versus dual-row fixation. *Arthroscopy* 2005;21:1307-1316.

80. Warner JJ, Tetreault P, Lehtinen J, Zurakowski D: Arthroscopic versus mini-open rotator cuff repair: A cohort comparison study. *Arthroscopy* 2005;21:328-332.

81. Youm T, Murray DH, Kubiak EN, Rokito AS, Zuckerman JD: Arthroscopic versus mini-open rotator cuff repair: A comparison of clinical outcomes and patient satisfaction. *J Shoulder Elbow Surg* 2005;14:455-459.

82. Prickett WD, Teefey SA, Galatz LM, Calfee RP, Middleton WD, Yamaguchi K: Accuracy of ultrasound imaging of the rotator cuff in shoulders that are painful postoperatively. *J Bone Joint Surg Am* 2003;85-A:1084-1089.

CHAPTER 3

SHOULDER INSTABILITY

WILLIAM N. LEVINE, MD
STEVEN S. GOLDBERG, MD

Arthroscopic treatment of shoulder instability was introduced in the 1980s as an alternative to open stabilization,[1] but early reports showed high rates of complications resulting from hardware problems, progression of arthritis, and recurrent subluxation.[2-4] As surgical techniques have advanced and indications for arthroscopic instability repair have become more clearly defined, the outcomes of these procedures have equaled or surpassed those of open stabilization. Arthroscopic treatment has the advantage of decreased soft-tissue morbidity and pain, less surgical time, improved cosmesis, and the ability to evaluate and treat coexisting pathology.[5] In this chapter we review the pathology of shoulder instability, describe the evaluation and indications for arthroscopic repair, discuss the current instrumentation and our preferred technique, and review the literature regarding arthroscopic treatment of shoulder instability.

PATHOLOGY OF INSTABILITY

The shoulder joint provides the greatest range of motion of any joint in the body and, therefore, is prone to the highest rate of dislocations. Because the joint has a shallow bony socket, stability depends largely on static and dynamic soft-tissue structures. Dynamic constraints, such as the rotator cuff, long head of the biceps, and scapular musculature, provide stability in the middle ranges of motion. Static constraints, such as the glenoid cartilage, labrum, and capsule, provide most of the stability at the end ranges of motion. The glenoid cartilage and labrum provide stability primarily by deepening the socket. The glenohumeral ligaments are thickenings of the joint capsule and serve as restraints to excessive humeral movement. The most important of these ligaments is the inferior glenohumeral ligament, the anterior band of which is the primary restraint to anterior glenohumeral translation while the arm is in abduction and external rotation, the position in which anterior dislocations usually occur.

Bankart described a separation of the anteroinferior labrum from the glenoid rim as the essential lesion in shoulder dislocations.[6] Subsequent studies have confirmed that this type of injury is the most common but not the only associated lesion. In one arthroscopic study of 212 patients with shoulder dislocations, an anterior glenoid labral tear was present in 87%, anterior capsule insufficiency in 79%, Hill-Sachs lesion in 68%, posterior glenohumeral ligament insufficiency in 55%, rotator cuff tears in 14%, and superior labral anterior and posterior (SLAP) lesions in 7%.[7] In another study limited to patients with traumatic dislocation, Bankart lesions occurred in 100% of shoulders.[8]

Although labral lesions affect socket depth and reduce the stability of the glenohumeral joint, biomechanical studies have clearly demonstrated that a Bankart lesion alone is insufficient to cause recurrent dislocation[9] and that plastic deformation of the capsule occurs.[10] Capsular injury may be difficult to assess during examination and arthroscopy, but failure to return the capsule to its proper tension often has been cited as a cause for failure of arthroscopic repair.[11]

The rotator interval is the space between the superior border of the subscapularis tendon and the anterior border of the supraspinatus tendon. The tendon of the long head of the biceps, portions of the superior and middle glenohumeral ligaments, and the coracohumeral ligament run in this space. Insufficiency of the rotator interval is associated with inferior instability, which may require arthroscopic closure of the interval.

Injury to the rotator cuff is more common after shoulder dislocation. Younger patients usually sustain partial undersurface tears of the supraspinatus that require no treatment, but patients older than age 40 years are at a much higher risk of full-thickness tears. Injuries to the superior labrum also should be identified because the biceps tendon provides stability by dynamic compression of the humeral head into the glenoid socket.[12]

PATIENT EVALUATION

History

The patient's history provides valuable information regarding the nature of the instability and associated pathology. Traumatic dislocations are likely to cause Bankart and Hill-Sachs lesions. Multidirectional instability (MDI) is suggested when shoulders dislocate with minimal trauma and in positions other than abduction and external rotation. For patients with multiple shoulder dislocations, it is important to distinguish recurrent anterior instability from MDI. Patients with recurrent anterior instability have poor results with nonsurgical treatment,[13] whereas those with MDI would benefit from a shoulder rehabilitation program before surgical treatment is attempted. Often the lines between these two groups are indistinct because instability lies along a wide spectrum, and even patients with traumatic dislocations have increased shoulder laxity on examination.

Physical Examination

A thorough examination is a necessary adjunct to the history. The examination must include assessment of neurovascular function including the axillary nerve, assessment of rotator cuff integrity, and testing for generalized ligamentous laxity. Specific instability tests are best performed with the patient supine. Recreating the patient's sensation of instability with the arm in abduction and external rotation indicates a positive apprehension test, and providing relief with a posteriorly applied force on the humerus indicates a positive relocation test. During the anterior release test, as the arm is brought into abduction and external rotation, the

FIGURE 1

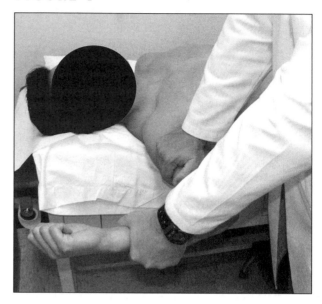

Clinical photograph of the anterior release test. The examiner's left hand is holding the patient's right arm. The examiner's right hand is reducing the anteriorly subluxated humeral head, and when it is released the shoulder will subluxate.

posterior force is removed rapidly and, if the test is positive, the patient has the feeling of instability[14] (Figure 1). Inferior laxity is assessed by applying downward traction with the arm in adduction and external rotation. A sulcus sign underneath the lateral acromion that is larger than 2 cm suggests rotator interval insufficiency. The posterior jerk test for posterior instability is performed with the arm in 90° forward flexion and maximal internal rotation. The examiner stabilizes the scapula with one hand while applying a posteriorly directed force to the patient's arm to elicit apprehension. O'Brien's active compression test is useful in identifying SLAP lesions.[15]

Radiographic Examination

Imaging should begin with plain radiographs and include an AP radiograph in the scapular plane and axillary radiographs to confirm a concentric glenohumeral joint and to identify associated fractures of the glenoid and humeral head. An AP radiograph with the arm in internal rotation best demonstrates Hill-Sachs compression fractures of the posterosuperior humeral head. A Stryker notch view also is useful for identifying Hill-Sachs lesions, whereas a West Point axillary view reliably visualizes bony Bankart lesions. MRI is excellent for evaluating the rotator cuff and other soft tissue, but MR arthrography is recommended for more accurate diagnosis of labral injury.[16]

INDICATIONS

Before capsular injury was recognized as a major factor in instability, recurrent dislocation after arthroscopic repair was common.[2-4] However, encouraging reports indicated that preservation of external rotation[17] and return to sporting activities[18] were reliable with arthroscopy. The problem likely was caused by surgeons addressing only the labral injury during arthroscopic repair rather than by a fault with the early devices. Results continued to improve as technologic advances allowed more secure tissue fixation and provided the ability to address both the capsule and the labrum. Older procedures using metallic staples and transglenoid sutures have been abandoned in favor of newer devices. Bioabsorbable single-point tacks are still used by some surgeons; however, the tacks are unable to address capsular laxity, and some patients have synovial reactions to the polyglyconate material. The most commonly used devices for treating instability are suture anchors.

Thermal capsulorrhaphy shrinks redundant glenohumeral capsular tissue by denaturing and shortening collagen molecules.[19] Although this technique received much initial interest,[20] long-term studies have shown a high rate of recurrent instability[21] and the potential for complications including capsular attenuation, axillary nerve injury,[22] and chondrolysis.[23]

Patients with traumatic anterior dislocations are the most common group of patients with instability and also are most likely to benefit from surgical intervention. In patients younger than age 20 years at initial dislocation, the reported rates of recurrence are as high as 90%.[24] The decision to acutely repair first-time dislocations should be made on an individual basis, but substantial evidence supports this approach.[25-27] First, the tissue is well vascularized and in good condition, making repair easier and healing more predictable. Second, further trauma to the anterior glenoid occurs with each dislocation, and the potential for significant alteration of the anterior bony morphology increases with recurrent dislocations.[28]

Relative contraindications to arthroscopic repair are large anterior bony defects, gross macroscopic lesions of the inferior glenohumeral ligament in the midsubstance, or avulsions of the glenohumeral ligament at the humeral insertion (HAGL lesions). Patients who engage in high-level contact sports are believed by some to be better served with open repair but this remains controversial.[18,29] However, a significant bony defect in a contact athlete represents a relative contraindication to arthroscopic repair.[30]

Patients with instability patterns other than anterior may be candidates for arthroscopic repair, provided the nature of the instability is clearly elicited during preoperative evaluation and examination under anesthesia (EUA), and all pathologic elements are addressed at the time of surgery. Patients with significant ligamentous laxity and MDI should be considered surgical candidates only after significant nonsurgical measures have been attempted. Arthroscopic capsular plication procedures have been described for patients with MDI, although the shift is glenoid-based. During biomechanical testing, both glenoid and humeral shifts had similar ability to reduce anterior and inferior translation.[31] Patients who voluntarily dislocate for secondary gain are poor candidates for any type of surgery.

TECHNIQUE

Setup

We prefer to perform arthroscopy on a patient under interscalene regional anesthesia in the beach chair or the lateral decubitus position. An adjustable pneumatic arm positioner is used with the beach chair position and holds the patient's limb in any position, obviating the need for an additional assistant.

Examination Under Anesthesia

Combining the information obtained from the history, physical examination, imaging, and EUA constitutes a complete preoperative evaluation of the patient with instability.

EUA allows the surgeon to assess the shoulder's laxity without patient guarding and is both highly sensitive and specific to findings at arthroscopy.[32] The load-and-shift test is performed with the arm in 20° of abduction, 20° of flexion, and neutral rotation. The

FIGURE 2

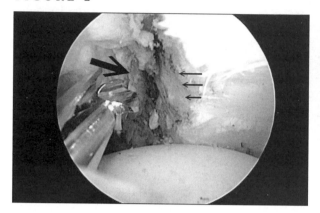

Arthroscopic view of the left shoulder through the anterosuperior portal. Large Bankart tear from 6 to 9 o'clock. The large black arrow points to the scapular neck after bony preparation. The three small black arrows point to the detached labral-ligamentous complex.

FIGURE 3

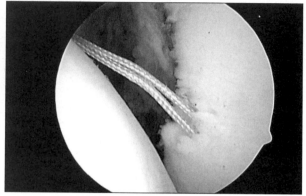

Arthroscopic view of the left shoulder through the posterior portal. The first suture anchor is placed as low as possible at the 6:30 o'clock position.

examiner holds the patient's proximal humerus with one hand while applying an axial load from the patient's elbow. Translation is assessed anteriorly, posteriorly, and inferiorly. Translation of the humerus is graded as follows: to the glenoid rim (1+), dislocation with spontaneous reduction (2+), and dislocation without spontaneous reduction (3+).[33]

Diagnostic Arthroscopy

The entire glenohumeral joint routinely is evaluated systematically. The integrity of the biceps anchor and superior labrum are checked. Although a sublabral foramen between the 12 and 3 o'clock positions is a normal variant,[34] any detachment below the glenoid equator is pathologic. The anterior band of the inferior glenohumeral ligament arises from the glenoid rim between the 3 and 5 o'clock positions. Rotator cuff tears, Hill-Sachs lesions, and HAGL lesions also must be identified. The anteroinferior glenoid may appear to be bare when the capsulolabral tissue is stripped from its origin and heals to the medial glenoid neck. Viewing from the anterosuperior portal will confirm this diagnosis. The anterior labral periosteal sleeve avulsion in which the anteroinferior glenoid appears bare requires mobilization of the tissue and repair back to the glenoid rim.[35]

The arthroscopic drive-through sign[36,37] is positive when the arthroscope easily can be passed through the joint from posterior to anterior at the level of the glenoid equator. This sign suggests capsular laxity but is not specific for anterior instability.

Portal Placement

Repair of the anteroinferior labrum requires establishing two anterior portals. The anterosuperior portal is established high within the rotator interval. Then the anteroinferior portal is established approximately 3 cm inferiorly at the skin level, entering the joint just above the rolled edge of the subscapularis. We prefer to establish portals in an outside-in technique using spinal needles to confirm placement.

Glenoid Preparation and Anchor Placement

The glenoid rim to which the labrum will be reattached is débrided of soft tissue and roughened using a rasp or shaver to expose a healthy bony surface (Figure 2). The labrum is freed and mobilized inferiorly to the 6 o'clock position or as far as the lesion extends. The first suture anchor is inserted at a 45° angle relative to the glenoid face from the anteroinferior portal and should be placed as inferiorly as possible, striving for the 5:30 o'clock position for the right shoulder or the 6:30 o'clock position for the left shoulder (Figure 3). The sutures are pulled on to ensure a solid fit of the anchor, and the scapula should lift off the table, confirming appropriate hold in the bone.

FIGURE 4

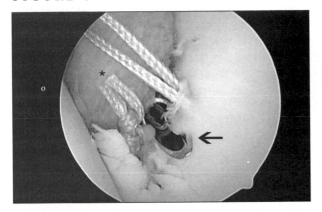

Arthroscopic view of the left shoulder through the posterior portal. SutureLasso tip (*arrow*) and nitinol wire are visualized after piercing the labral-ligamentous tissue (asterisk) just inferior to the second suture anchor, which is at the 8 o'clock position.

FIGURE 5

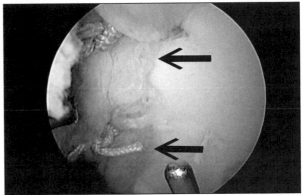

Arthroscopic view of the left shoulder through the anterosuperior portal. Final repair after three suture anchors are placed and the sutures are tied. Large black arrows point to the articular cartilage-labrum junction, showing the recreation of the normal anatomic relationship.

Suture Management and Knot Tying

One limb of the suture pair is retrieved through the anterosuperior portal to simplify suture management. A variety of passing devices are available, and it is useful to have several in the operating room. We typically use the SutureLasso (Arthrex, Naples, FL) shuttle system, introduced from the anteroinferior portal. The capsule and labrum should be pierced inferior to the anchor location to shift the capsule superiorly and reestablish normal tension (Figure 4). Once the instrument has passed through the tissue and the tip is visible, the thin wire loop is advanced and retrieved through the anterosuperior portal using the suture grasper. The suture shuttle is removed, leaving only the wire loop in the tissue. The suture limb from the anterosuperior portal is placed through the wire loop and both are pulled back out of the anteroinferior portal, passing that limb of the suture through the capsule and labrum. This suture limb will be the post during tying to keep the knot as far as possible from the articular surface.

We prefer a Tennessee slider knot because of its ease in tying, low bulk, and reproducibility. However, there are many other excellent knot choices. More important than the choice of knot is proper knot-tying technique,[38] which involves maintaining tension on the post (loop security) to compress the knot down on the tissue. Good technique also involves tying alternating half hitches that

lie flat and do not slip under normal load conditions (knot security). Once the first anchor is placed, sequential anchors are placed superiorly in a similar manner, with the end result recreating the normal labral bumper (Figure 5). Typically this requires three anchors but more may be necessary. Moving the camera to the anterosuperior portal during the repair affords good visualization of the anterior glenoid. The final repair should be confirmed from the anterior portal.

Rotator Interval Closure and Capsular Plication

After capsule and labral repair are completed, other structures (rotator cuff, rotator interval, SLAP lesion) are repaired as necessary. The rotator interval is closed with a suture placed through the capsule, just above the rolled edge of the subscapularis and just anterior to the supraspinatus. Care should be taken to not overtighten the rotator interval.

Capsular plication may be performed in the inferior pouch if excessive volume remains after the labrum is repaired. This procedure involves passing the suture through the capsule, advancing it to the labrum, and closing down the volume of the inferior pouch. If all sources of laxity are addressed, the drive-through sign should no longer be positive. We do not perform thermal capsulorrhaphy because its long-term success has not been established, and complications can be severe.

Rehabilitation

The patient's arm is placed in a sling, and pendulum exercises are started immediately. Patients are referred for physical therapy starting in the second week after surgery. Passive and active exercises are begun with limits of range of motion determined by intraoperative and patient-specific guidelines. The goal is to achieve full range of motion by 6 to 8 weeks. Mild resistance exercises are initiated at 6 to 10 weeks. Strengthening exercises are started after week 10, and return to sport usually is allowed after 4 to 6 months.

COMPLICATIONS

Although complications after this procedure are infrequent, they must be recognized. Injury to the axillary nerve can occur because it travels only an average of 2.5 mm deep to the inferior glenohumeral ligament and lies only 12 mm from the glenoid at the 6 o'clock position.[39] Axillary nerve injury has been reported more commonly after thermal capsulorrhaphy, typically involves sensory function only, and usually recovers spontaneously.[22] Recurrent dislocations may result from insufficient restoration of normal capsular anatomy or failure to recognize other concurrent pathology. Arthroscopic repairs may not be successful in shoulders with large bony glenoid defects[30,40] or in shoulders with large Hill-Sachs compression fractures. A large Hill-Sachs lesion may engage the glenoid surface in abduction and external rotation and give the sensation of recurrent instability. This lesion also effectively reduces the humeral arc of motion because of its location on the posterior articular surface.[41]

RESULTS OF ARTHROSCOPIC REPAIR

For first-time traumatic dislocations, arthroscopic repair dramatically decreases the rate of recurrence compared with nonsurgical treatment.[25-27] Bottoni and associates[27] reported an 11% rate of recurrence after arthroscopic stabilization compared with 75% after nonsurgical treatment. Kirkley and associates[26] showed a threefold reduction in redislocation and demonstrated objective improvement in disease-specific quality-of-life measurements with arthroscopic repair.

Similarly good results for both groups have been reported in several studies directly comparing arthroscopic and open techniques.[42-44] The success rate of arthroscopic repair in highly active patients approaches or exceeds 90% in several studies.[18,25,45] Good or excellent results were achieved at 2- to 6-year follow-up in 95% of a series of 167 patients in whom modern suture anchors were used. The mean loss of external rotation was only 2°, and 91% of the patients returned to near or equal their preinjury level. A glenoid defect larger than 30% of glenoid circumference was strongly associated with recurrent instability.[40]

For anterior and inferior instability, the best results have been obtained when all lesions were addressed at surgery. Gartsman and associates[46] reported 92% good or excellent results and return to sports in 89%, concluding that appropriate capsule tensioning and rotator interval closure were important in achieving these results. For patients with inferior instability and no other defects, isolated rotator interval closure has been successful.[47]

Good results also were reported for arthroscopic treatment of traumatic posterior instability.[48-50] Arthroscopic treatment also may be a viable option for patients with MDI resistant to nonsurgical treatment.[51,52] Results of an arthroscopic capsular plication procedure were reported by Treacy and associates,[53] who achieved 88% satisfactory results by Neer's criteria, which is comparable with the results of the open inferior capsular shift.

SUMMARY

As techniques have evolved, the ability to treat instability using all arthroscopic methods has improved, with results equaling or exceeding those of open procedures. Patients with traumatic anterior and inferior dislocations, those with MDI, and even athletes may be treated arthroscopically with success. The key to optimizing outcomes lies in identifying patients who are not good candidates for arthroscopic repair—patients with large bony glenoid defects or large humeral head defects (Hill-Sachs lesions), capsular tears, and HAGL lesions. Success also lies in treating all pathologic findings at surgery, not just the Bankart lesion. The synthesis of information gathered during a thorough history, careful physical examination, and EUA will allow the surgeon to address all the needs of the patient with an unstable shoulder.

REFERENCES

1. Matthews LS, Vetter WL, Oweida SJ, Spearman J, Helfet DL: Arthroscopic staple capsulorrhaphy for recurrent anterior shoulder instability. *Arthroscopy* 1988;4:106-111.

2. Guanche CA, Quick DC, Sodergren KM, Buss DD: Arthroscopic versus open reconstruction of the shoulder in patients with isolated Bankart lesions. *Am J Sports Med* 1996;24:144-148.

3. Freedman KB, Smith AP, Romeo AA, Cole BJ, Bach BR Jr: Open Bankart repair versus arthroscopic repair with transglenoid sutures or bioabsorbable tacks for recurrent anterior instability of the shoulder: A meta-analysis. *Am J Sports Med* 2004;32:1520-1527.

4. Sperber A, Hamberg P, Karlsson J, Sward L, Wredmark T: Comparison of an arthroscopic and an open procedure for posttraumatic instability of the shoulder: A prospective, randomized multicenter study. *J Shoulder Elbow Surg* 2001;10:105-108.

5. Cole BJ, Warner JJP: Arthroscopic anterior glenohumeral ligament reconstruction, in Norris TR (ed): *Orthopaedic Knowledge Update: Shoulder and Elbow 2.* Rosemont, IL, American Academy of Orthopaedic Surgeons, 2002, pp 103-115.

6. Bankart A: The pathology and treatment of recurrent dislocation of the shoulder-joint. *Br J Surg* 1938;26:23-29.

7. Hintermann B, Gachter A: Arthroscopic findings after shoulder dislocation. *Am J Sports Med* 1995;23:545-551.

8. Norlin R: Intraarticular pathology in acute, first-time anterior shoulder dislocation: An arthroscopic study. *Arthroscopy* 1993;9:546-549.

9. Speer KP, Deng X, Borrero S, Torzilli PA, Altchek DA, Warren RF: Biomechanical evaluation of a simulated Bankart lesion. *J Bone Joint Surg Am* 1994;76:1819-1826.

10. Bigliani LU, Pollock RG, Soslowsky LJ, Flatow EL, Pawluk RJ, Mow VC: Tensile properties of the inferior glenohumeral ligament. *J Orthop Res* 1992;10:187-197.

11. Mologne TS, McBride MT, Lapoint JM: Assessment of failed arthroscopic anterior labral repairs: Findings at open surgery. *Am J Sports Med* 1997;25:813-817.

12. Lippitt SB, Vanderhooft JE, Harris SL, Sidles J, Harryman D, Matsen F: Glenohumeral stability from concavity-compression: A quantitative analysis. *J Shoulder Elbow Surg* 1993;2:27-35.

13. Burkhead WZ Jr, Rockwood CA Jr: Treatment of instability of the shoulder with an exercise program. *J Bone Joint Surg Am* 1992;74:890-896.

14. Gross ML, Distefano MC: Anterior release test: A new test for occult shoulder instability. *Clin Orthop Relat Res* 1997;339:105-108.

15. O'Brien SJ, Pagnani MJ, Fealy S, McGlynn SR, Wilson JB: The active compression test: A new and effective test for diagnosing labral tears and acromioclavicular joint abnormality. *Am J Sports Med* 1998;26:610-613.

16. Parmar H, Jhankaria B, Maheshwari M, et al: Magnetic resonance arthrography in recurrent anterior shoulder instability as compared to arthroscopy: A prospective comparative study. *J Postgrad Med* 2002;48:270-273.

17. Karlsson J, Magnusson L, Ejerhed L, Hultenheim I, Lundin O, Kartus J: Comparison of open and arthroscopic stabilization for recurrent shoulder dislocation in patients with a Bankart lesion. *Am J Sports Med* 2001;29:538-542.

18. Bacilla P, Field LD, Savoie FH III: Arthroscopic Bankart repair in a high demand patient population. *Arthroscopy* 1997;13:51-60.

19. Wall MS, Deng XH, Torzilli PA, Doty SB, O'Brien SJ, Warren RF: Thermal modification of collagen. *J Shoulder Elbow Surg* 1999;8:339-344.

20. Hawkins RJ, Karas SG: Arthroscopic stabilization plus thermal capsulorrhaphy for anterior instability with and without Bankart lesions: The role of rehabilitation and immobilization. *Instr Course Lect* 2001;50:13-15.

21. D'Alessandro DF, Bradley JP, Fleischli JE, Connor PM: Prospective evaluation of thermal capsulorrhaphy for shoulder instability: Indications and results, two- to five-year follow-up. *Am J Sports Med* 2004;32:21-33.

22. Wong KL, Williams GR: Complications of thermal capsulorrhaphy of the shoulder. *J Bone Joint Surg Am* 2001;83(suppl 2):151-155.

23. Levine WN, Clark AM, D'Alessandro DF, Yamaguchi K: Chondrolysis following arthroscopic thermal capsulorrhaphy to treat shoulder instability: A report of two cases. *J Bone Joint Surg Am* 2005;87:616-621.

24. Hovelius L: Shoulder dislocation in Swedish ice hockey players. *Am J Sports Med* 1978;6:373-377.

25. DeBerardino TM, Arciero RA, Taylor DC, Uhorchak JM: Prospective evaluation of arthroscopic stabilization of acute, initial anterior shoulder dislocations in young athletes: Two- to five-year follow-up. *Am J Sports Med* 2001;29:586-592.

26. Kirkley A, Griffin S, Richards C, Miniaci A, Mohtadi N: Prospective randomized clinical trial comparing the effectiveness of immediate arthroscopic stabilization versus immobilization and rehabilitation in first traumatic anterior dislocations of the shoulder. *Arthroscopy* 1999;15:507-514.

27. Bottoni CR, Wilckens JH, DeBerardino TM, et al: A prospective, randomized evaluation of arthroscopic sta-

bilization versus nonoperative treatment in patients with acute, traumatic, first-time shoulder dislocations. *Am J Sports Med* 2002;30:576-580.

28. Hunter RE: The role of arthroscopy for acute shoulder dislocations, in Norris TR (ed): *Orthopaedic Knowledge Update: Shoulder and Elbow 2.* Rosemont, IL, American Academy of Orthopaedic Surgeons, 2002, pp 487-493.

29. Grana WA, Buckley PD, Yates CK: Arthroscopic Bankart suture repair. *Am J Sports Med* 1993;21:348-353.

30. Burkhart SS, De Beer JF: Traumatic glenohumeral bone defects and their relationship to failure of arthroscopic Bankart repairs: Significance of the inverted-pear glenoid and the humeral engaging Hill-Sachs lesion. *Arthroscopy* 2000;16:677-694.

31. Deutsch A, Barber JE, Davy DT, Victoroff BN: Anterior-inferior capsular shift of the shoulder: A biomechanical comparison of glenoid-based versus humeral-based shift strategies. *J Shoulder Elbow Surg* 2001;10:340-352.

32. Cofield RH, Nessler JP, Weinstabl R: Diagnosis of shoulder instability by examination under anesthesia. *Clin Orthop Relat Res* 1993;291:45-53.

33. Hawkins RJ, Schutte JP, Janda DH, Huckell GH: Translation of the glenohumeral joint with the patient under anesthesia. *J Shoulder Elbow Surg* 1996;5:286-292.

34. Ilahi OA, Labbe MR, Cosculluela P: Variants of the anterosuperior glenoid labrum and associated pathology. *Arthroscopy* 2002;18:882-886.

35. Neviaser TJ: The anterior labroligamentous periosteal sleeve avulsion lesion: A cause of anterior instability of the shoulder. *Arthroscopy* 1993;9:17-21.

36. McFarland EG, Neira CA, Gutierrez MI, Cosgarea AJ, Magee M: Clinical significance of the arthroscopic drive-through sign in shoulder surgery. *Arthroscopy* 2001;17:38-43.

37. Pagnani MJ, Warren RF, Altchek DW, Wickiewicz TL, Anderson AF: Arthroscopic shoulder stabilization using transglenoid sutures: Four-year minimum followup. *Am J Sports Med* 1996;24:459-467.

38. Lo IK, Burkhart SS, Chan KC, Athanasiou K: Arthroscopic knots: Determining the optimal balance of loop security and knot security. *Arthroscopy* 2004;20:489-502.

39. Price MR, Tillett ED, Acland RD, Nettleton GS: Determining the relationship of the axillary nerve to the shoulder joint capsule from an arthroscopic perspective. *J Bone Joint Surg Am* 2004;86:2135-2142.

40. Kim SH, Ha KI, Cho YB, Ryu BD, Oh I: Arthroscopic anterior stabilization of the shoulder: Two to six-year follow-up. *J Bone Joint Surg Am* 2003;85:1511-1518.

41. Burkhart SS, Danaceau SM: Articular arc length mismatch as a cause of failed bankart repair. *Arthroscopy* 2000;16:740-744.

42. Fabbriciani C, Milano G, Demontis A, Fadda S, Ziranu F, Mulas PD: Arthroscopic versus open treatment of Bankart lesion of the shoulder: A prospective randomized study. *Arthroscopy* 2004;20:456-462.

43. Kim SH, Ha KI, Kim SH: Bankart repair in traumatic anterior shoulder instability: Open versus arthroscopic technique. *Arthroscopy* 2002;18:755-763.

44. Cole BJ, L'Insalata J, Irrgang J, Warner JJ: Comparison of arthroscopic and open anterior shoulder stabilization: A two to six-year follow-up study. *J Bone Joint Surg Am* 2000;82:1108-1114.

45. Porcellini G, Campi F, Paladini P: Arthroscopic approach to acute bony Bankart lesion. *Arthroscopy* 2002;18:764-769.

46. Gartsman GM, Roddey TS, Hammerman SM: Arthroscopic treatment of anterior-inferior glenohumeral instability: Two to five-year follow-up. *J Bone Joint Surg Am* 2000;82:991-1003.

47. Field LD, et al: Isolated closure of rotator interval defects for shoulder instability. *Am J SportsMed* 1995;23:557-563.

48. Williams RJ III, Strickland S, Cohen M, Altchek DW, Warren RF: Arthroscopic repair for traumatic posterior shoulder instability. *Am J Sports Med* 2003;31:203-209.

49. McIntyre LF, Caspari RB, Savoie FH III: The arthroscopic treatment of posterior shoulder instability: Two-year results of a multiple suture technique. *Arthroscopy* 1997;13:426-432.

50. Antoniou J, Duckworth DT, Harryman DT II: Capsulolabral augmentation for the the management of posteroinferior instability of the shoulder. *J Bone Joint Surg Am* 2000;82:1220-1230.

51. McIntyre LF, Caspari RB, Savoie FH III: The arthroscopic treatment of multidirectional shoulder instability: Two-year results of a multiple suture technique. *Arthroscopy* 1997;13:418-425.

52. Hewitt M, Getelman MH, Snyder SJ: Arthroscopic management of multidirectional instability: Pancapsular plication. *Orthop Clin North Am* 2003;34:549-557.

53. Treacy SH, Savoie FH III, Field LD: Arthroscopic treatment of multidirectional instability. *J Shoulder Elbow Surg* 1999;8:345-350.

CHAPTER 4

SLAP Lesions and Disorders of the Long Head of the Biceps

CHRISTOPHER S. AHMAD, MD
NEAL S. ELATTRACHE, MD

INTRODUCTION

The term SLAP (superior labral anterior and posterior) lesions has been used to describe injuries to the superior labrum.[1] These lesions recently have been recognized as a significant cause of shoulder pain. Recent literature has established consistent features from the history and physical examination, which are complemented by advances in MRI, to assist accurate diagnosis. Arthroscopic procedures to repair these injuries also have evolved and proven effective.

Proximal long head of the biceps disorders that are independent of SLAP lesions are also common and can be a source of pain and disability. Strategies are being developed to treat specific long head of the biceps disorders with either débridement, tenotomy, or tenodesis. This chapter reviews the anatomy, biomechanics, classification, diagnosis, and current treatment recommendations for SLAP lesions and long head of the biceps tendon disorders.

ANATOMY

Thorough knowledge of the normal anatomy of the superior labrum and biceps is critical to proper recognition of abnormal pathology. Although the labrum, located directly anterior, posterior, and inferior to the glenoid, is a consistent rounded fibrous structure continuous with the articular cartilage, the superior labrum has a high degree of normal variation. It may be rounded or have a meniscus-type appearance, with the meniscal component overlying but not attached to the glenoid articular surface (Figure 1). In a recent series, 49 of 191 patients were reported on arthroscopic examination to have a mobile meniscoid-type superior labrum, which was treated with observation. That only one of these patients became clinically symptomatic emphasizes the importance of proper recognition of this anatomy and of avoiding inappropriate fixation.[2] The Buford complex, is a normal variant, consisting of a cord-like middle glenohumeral ligament (MGHL) that originates directly from the superior labrum at the base of the biceps tendon with absence of anterosuperior labral tissue (Figure 2). The sublabral foramen is a cord-like MGHL with a direct attachment to the anterosuperior labrum that creates a hole between the ligament and the glenoid. Inappropriate attachment of the cord-like MGHL to this void on the anterosuperior glenoid results in painful restriction of external rotation and elevation. The presence of a cord-like MGHL in isolation (18%) is more common than its presence in combination with the Buford complex (1% to 2%).[3,4]

BIOMECHANICS

The overall labrum adds stability to the glenohumeral joint by providing depth and surface area to the glenoid.[5,6] The function of the long head of the biceps tendon remains controversial. Biomechanical studies suggests the biceps tendon functions as a dynamic stabilizer to the anterior stability of the glenohumeral joint.[7,8] Recently, Burkart and associates[9] reported that repair of a type II SLAP lesion restored greater glenohumeral stability to inferior translation than to anterior translation. Data from other studies, using electromyography, suggest that the biceps muscle is active with

FIGURE 1

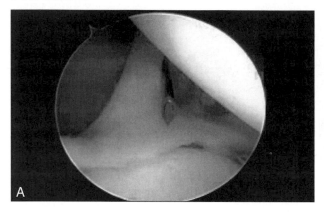

Normal superior labrum morphology. **A,** Meniscoid type **B,** Rounded type.

elbow function only.[10,11] In another recent biomechanical study, isolated lesions of the anterosuperior portion of the labrum, which did not involve the long head of the biceps, had no significant effect on anteroposterior or superoinferior glenohumeral translation, whereas complete lesions of the superior labrum and biceps insertion resulted in significant increases in glenohumeral translation instability.[12]

Biomechanical studies also have been used to investigate the mechanism by which SLAP injuries are created. Bey and associates[13] reported that traction on the biceps tendon can reproducibly create type II SLAP lesions if the glenohumeral joint is subluxated inferiorly. Clavert and associates[14] simulated falls forward and backward; they reported production of more type II SLAP lesions with forward falls and attributed the development of these lesions to shearing forces. Kuhn and associates[15] studied the throwing motion and reported that SLAP lesions occurred more commonly in the late cocking position than in the early deceleration position.

SLAP LESIONS

Classification

Snyder and associates[1] originally described four types of SLAP lesions. Type I lesions consist of fraying and degeneration of the superior labrum without instability of the long head of the biceps attachment (Figure 3, *A*). Type II lesions consist of detachment of the biceps tendon anchor from the superior glenoid tubercle (Figure

FIGURE 2

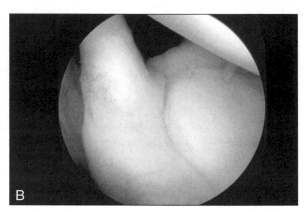

Biceps tendon

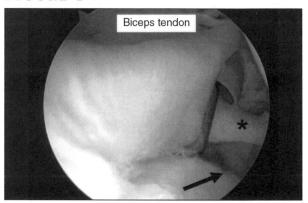

Buford complex demonstrating cord-like MGHL (asterisk) behind the probe originating adjacent to the biceps. Arrow indicates sublabral foramen.

3, *B*). Morgan and associates[16] subclassified type II SLAP lesions into (1) anterior, (2) posterior, and (3) combined anterior and posterior lesions. Type III lesions (Figure 3, *C*) consist of a bucket handle tear of a meniscoid superior labrum with an intact biceps tendon anchor, and type IV lesions (Figure 3, *D*) consist of a superior labral tear that extends into the biceps tendon. Kim and associates[17] recently reported that 74% of the SLAP lesions were type I, 21% were type II, 0.7% were type III, and 4% were type IV. In addition, most of the SLAP lesions (123 of 139) were reported to be associated with other intra-articular lesions.

Some SLAP lesions are a combination of the lesions described above. Most often, these are type III or IV

FIGURE 3

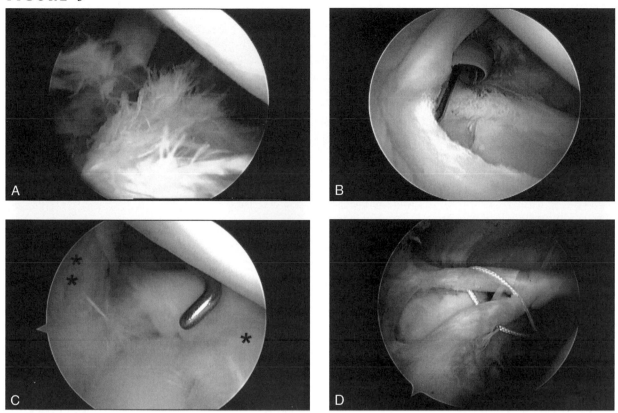

Classification of SLAP lesions. **A,** Type I with frayed labrum and intact biceps anchor. **B,** Type II with probe demonstrating unstable biceps anchor. **C,** Type III, asterisk indicates inferiorly displaced labrum, and double asterisk indicates biceps tendon. **D,** Type IV.

lesions combined with a significantly detached biceps anchor (type II lesions). These lesions are classified as complex SLAP lesions type II and III or type II and IV. Maffet and associates[18] expanded this classification to include (1) anteroinferior Bankart-type labral lesions in continuity with SLAP lesions, (2) biceps tendon separation with an unstable flap tear of the labrum, and (3) extension of the superior labrum-biceps tendon separation to beneath the MGHL.

Diagnosis

History

The mechanism of injury is either acute shoulder traction or compression or repetitive overhead activity. Anterior traction injuries result from sports such as water skiing; superior traction injuries result from attempting to break a fall from a height; and inferior traction injuries result from a sudden inferior pull.[1,18] Compression of the glenohumeral joint as a result of a fall onto an outstretched hand in forward flexion and abduction or a direct blow to the glenohumeral joint cause an impaction injury of the humeral head against the superior labrum and the biceps anchor.[1,19,20] A type II lesion results when the biceps tendon is avulsed from the superior glenoid as it is tensioned over the humeral head. If a meniscoid-type superior labrum is present, a type III or IV lesion may result, with the formation of a bucket handle fragment.

Throwing or overhead motions can create SLAP lesions by traction to the biceps anchor with humeral rotation. Andrews and associates[21] first observed anterosuperior glenoid labrum tears in throwers and postulated a traction injury that occurred in the follow-through phase of throwing, with the biceps acting as a decelerator of the rapidly extending elbow.

Burkhart and Morgan[22] described a peel-back mechanism that consists of torsional force imposed on the biceps during late cocking; this mechanism can be reproduced during an arthroscopic examination.

Symptoms include anterosuperior or posterosuperior shoulder pain exacerbated by activity with the arm overhead. Popping, locking, and snapping may occur with unstable labral tears. Instability symptoms may be present if the tear extends into the anterior ligament and labrum, resulting in a Bankart lesion.

Physical Examination

Many tests have been described that assist in diagnosing SLAP lesions. The active compression test has good correlation for type II SLAP lesions.[23] The arm is positioned in 20° of adduction and 90° of forward elevation. The examiner applies downward force on the forearm while the hand is both pronated and supinated and compares the resulting pain and weakness. A positive test occurs when the patient reports pain that is worse in the pronated position. The compression-rotation test is similar to McMurray's test of the knee.[24] It is performed by compressing the glenohumeral joint and then rotating the humerus in an attempt to trap the labrum in the joint. This test should be performed with the patient in the supine position, where he or she is more relaxed.

Speed's biceps tension test is sensitive for SLAP lesions.[19,20] This test is performed by having the patient resist downward pressure with his or her arm in 90° of forward elevation with the elbow extended and the forearm supinated. Although this test is more suggestive of biceps tendon damage, it reproduces symptoms with an unstable anchor. A positive apprehension relocation sign for posterior shoulder pain may suggest a SLAP lesion in the posterior labrum as part of a spectrum of internal impingement.

Many other tests have been described, including the biceps load test II,[25] anterior slide test,[26] and pain provocation test,[27] but we have found them to be less useful. Studies investigating the diagnostic accuracy of many of these tests have resulted in controversy regarding their individual sensitivity and specificity. In a recent study, subjects underwent Speed's test, Yergason's test, the O'Brien active compression test, the anterior apprehension test, the Jobe relocation test, the crank test, and a test for tenderness of the bicipital groove.[28] The examination results were compared with surgical findings and analyzed for sensitivity and specificity in the diagnosis

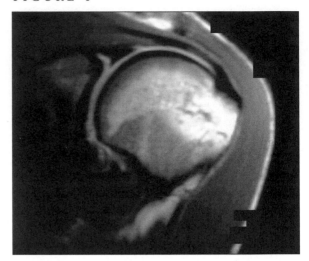

FIGURE 4

Gadolinium-enhanced coronal oblique MRI scan with dye under the biceps anchor indicating type II SLAP tear.

of SLAP lesions and other glenoid labral tears. The results of the O'Brien test (63% sensitive, 73% specific) and the Jobe relocation test (44% sensitive, 87% specific) were statistically correlated with the presence of a tear in the labrum, and the apprehension test approached statistical significance. Performing all three tests and accepting a positive result for any of them increased the statistical value, although the sensitivity and specificity were still disappointingly low (72% and 73%, respectively). The other four tests were not found to be useful for labral tears, and none of the tests or combinations were statistically valid for specific detection of a SLAP lesion.

Imaging

Radiographic evaluation includes the standard three views of the shoulder (AP, axillary, and outlet views). These radiographs do not assist in evaluating for SLAP lesion but help exclude other potential abnormalities. MR arthrography has been demonstrated to be superior to plain MRI for diagnosing SLAP lesions.[29] Bencardino and associates[29] reported a sensitivity of 89%, a specificity of 91%, and an accuracy of 90% in detecting labral lesions. The main MRI feature is the presence of contrast between the superior labrum and the glenoid that extends well around and below the biceps anchor on the coronal oblique view (Figure 4). Often, contrast will diffuse into the labral fragment, causing it to appear ragged or indistinct. The axial views visualize possible extention into the anterior and or posterior labrum. Normal labral variants, such as a cordlike MGHL and sublabral foramen, must be differentiated from anterosuperior labral pathology.

Arthroscopic Evaluation

Although history, physical examination, and MRI can provide useful information in the diagnosis of SLAP lesions, the ultimate diagnosis relies on arthroscopic evaluation.[30] Types I, III, and IV lesions are obvious when fraying or splitting of the labrum is noted. Viewing from both the anterior and posterior portals is mandatory to assess the entire degree of involvement. Diagnosis of type II lesions is more difficult. The normal superior labrum often has a small cleft between it and the glenoid, especially in the setting of a meniscoid labrum; therefore, the stability of the biceps anchor is determined by probing and attempting to elevate the labrum and biceps. The glenoid articular cartilage usually extends medially over the superior corner of the glenoid, and absence of cartilage indicates detachment. Traction on the biceps tendon will demonstrate any loss of integrity at the labral attachment and instability of the attached ligaments. Burkhart and Morgan[22] have described arthroscopic examination for peel back in which the arm is removed from traction and placed in a throwing position. As the abducted humerus is rotated from internal to external rotation, the labrum peels away from the posterosuperior glenoid.

Treatment

Nonsurgical Management

The role of nonsurgical management of unstable SLAP lesions remains controversial. Snyder and associates[20] have argued that nonsurgical treatment generally yields poor results, although few studies are directed at nonsurgical treatment and the natural history of the lesions. In one study, patients had an extended trial of activity modification and rehabilitation exercises.[12] Most patients had been treated with rest, physical therapy, steroid injections, and nonsteroidal anti-inflammatory drugs (NSAIDs) without relief of their symptoms before diagnostic arthroscopy.

For patients with an acute shoulder injury, initial treatment is directed at eliminating pain, restoring motion, correcting strength deficits, and restoring normal synchronous muscle activity. Pain is eliminated by instituting rest, avoidance of the aggravating activities, a course of NSAIDs, cryotherapy, and other therapeutic measures. Aggressive strengthening is initiated once pain is resolved. For throwing athletes, a gradual return to throwing may begin as muscular balance and range of motion are restored. Failure of a nonsurgical program, early suspicion of significant mechanical dysfunction, or seasonal timing may direct treatment toward surgical intervention.

Surgical Management

Type I SLAP lesions are treated with débridement; type II SLAP lesions are repaired using a suture anchor technique for fixation; and type III SLAP lesions are treated by resection of the unstable bucket handle labral fragment for small detachments. For larger tears, repair may be preferred. Type IV SLAP lesions are treated similarly to type III lesions unless the biceps tendon split is severe. The tendon is managed with either release, repair as with a type II SLAP lesion, or biceps tenodesis. The decision depends on the age and activity level of the patient and the condition of the remainder of the biceps tendon.

SLAP Lesion Repair Technique

SLAP lesion repairs may be performed with the patient in the beach chair or lateral decubitus position. We prefer the lateral decubitus position. A posterior viewing portal is established, and the biceps-superior labral complex is evaluated. A spinal needle introduced anteriorly may be used to probe the superior labrum before committing to the location of the anterior portal. Proper placement of the suture anchors requires exact placement of the anterosuperior portal in the superior aspect of the rotator interval and slightly superior to the biceps tendon. A cannula is placed, and a probe is used to test the stability of the biceps and superior labrum attachments to the glenoid (Figure 3, B) To perform the peelback test, the arm is positioned to 90° abduction and 90° external rotation. Existence of a posterior SLAP lesion will cause the biceps-superior labrum complex to drop medially over the edge of the glenoid.

After confirming the presence of a reparable lesion, a motorized shaver from the anterior working portal is used to prepare the superior neck of the glenoid beneath the detached labrum (Figure 5). The soft tissues are débrided, and the bone is abraded to enhance healing.

FIGURE 5

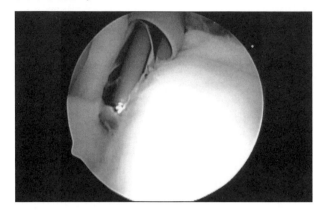

Shaver used to débride superior glenoid.

FIGURE 6

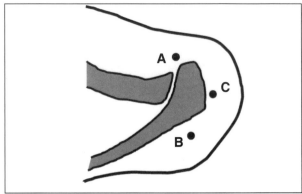

A, Anterior working portal. **B,** Standard viewing portal. **C,** Wilmington portal located adjacent to acromion in posterior third.

FIGURE 7

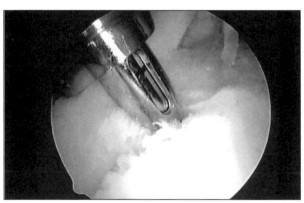

Guide for suture anchor placement introduced through the Wilmington portal.

FIGURE 8

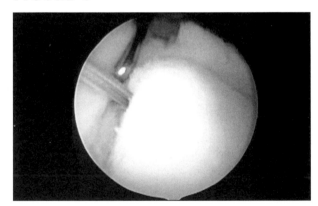

Suture anchor location is confirmed to be in bone and adjacent to articular cartilage.

A Wilmington portal is placed at the lateral edge of the acromion at its posterior one third (Figure 6). A suture anchor is placed through this cannula adjacent to the biceps tendon at the glenoid margin (Figure 7). The suture anchor must be visualized and confirmed to be in bone, and it must be tested with tension to confirm it is secure (Figure 8). Next, the suture is passed through the labrum using the device chosen by the surgeon from among the several available devices. The most popular devices are instruments that penetrate the labrum from superior to inferior, which allows grasping of the suture. This technique avoids suture shuttling. An alternative technique is to use a suture-passing device that requires suture shuttling. The limb of the suture facing the labrum is retrieved out of the anterior portal. The suture-passing device is passed through the labrum, and the suture shuttle is retrieved out of the anterior portal (Figure 9). The suture is then shuttled through the labrum and to the posterior cannula. Arthroscopic knot tying is then performed. A probe is used to assess the repair. The process of anchor placement, suture passing, and knot tying is repeated anteriorly and posteriorly as needed (Figure 10).

Postoperative Protocol

Postoperatively, the shoulder is protected in a sling for 3 to 6 weeks. The patient begins elbow, wrist, and hand

FIGURE 9

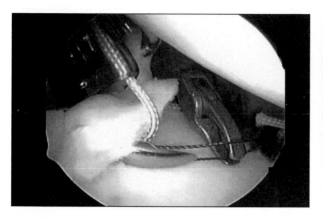

Suture passer placed through the labrum with wire shuttle being retrieved out anterior portal.

FIGURE 10

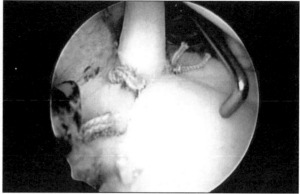

Completed repair with several anchors placed and knots tied.

exercises immediately postoperatively and gentle pendulum exercises in 1 week. The shoulder is protected to avoid stress on the biceps tendon for 6 weeks. Strengthening exercises for the rotator cuff, scapular stabilizers, and deltoid are initiated with restoration of range of motion at 6 weeks, and biceps strengthening is begun 8 weeks postoperatively. Vigorous or strenuous lifting activities are allowed after 3 months. At 4 months, throwing athletes begin an interval throwing program on a level surface. They continue a stretching and strengthening program, with particular emphasis on posteroinferior capsular stretching. At 6 months, pitchers may begin throwing full-speed, and at 7 months pitchers are allowed maximal effort throwing from the mound.

Outcomes

Simple débridement has been shown to yield poor results for unstable SLAP lesions.[31] Surgical repair has achieved improved results as fixation techniques have evolved. Stapling[32] and bioabsorbable tac[20,33-35] devices were introduced with improved outcomes compared with débridment alone. There have been concerns regarding synovitis, foreign body reaction, adhesive capsulitis, and breakage of the tac devices.[20,34,36,37]

Transglenoid sutures also have been used to repair SLAP lesions with good results, but they involve substantial technical difficulty.[19] In more recent studies, suture anchor fixation has been used with good and excellent results.[16,38-40] Kim and associates[39] reported repair with suture anchors in 34 patients with isolated SLAP lesions, with 94% satisfactory results; 91% regained their preinjury level of shoulder function. Morgan and associates[16] reported on throwing athletes with an 87% return to preinjury levels of throwing.

PATHOLOGY ISOLATED TO THE LONG HEAD OF THE BICEPS

Biceps instability and biceps tendinitis are common disorders of the long head of the biceps that are independent of SLAP lesions.[41] Mechanical impingement of the biceps tendon against the coracoacromial arch, which is similar to rotator cuff impingement, has been described as a cause of biceps degeneration.[42-45] The degenerative process causes atrophy of the tendon or the impingement results in chronic inflammation that causes hypertrophy.[11] The loss of soft-tissue restraints, which often is associated with rotator cuff tears, results in subluxation of the long head of the biceps.[46-49] Medial subluxation of the long head of the biceps occurs most often in the presence of a subscapularis tear.[41]

Diagnosis

History

Pain is localized to the anterolateral aspects of the shoulder and radiates into the biceps muscle.[46-48,50]

FIGURE 11

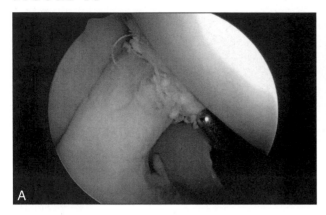 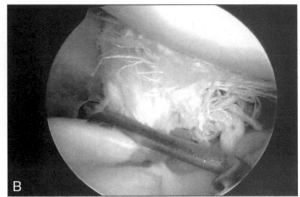

Arthroscopic view of long head of biceps tendon within the glenohumeral joint. **A,** More normal appearance before drawing the tendon into the joint. **B,** Significant degeneration of the tendon after drawing the tendon into the joint with the probe.

Concomitant rotator cuff disorders may add to the pain. Painful snapping or clicking in the shoulder, usually with the arm in an overhead position with internal to external humeral rotation, occurs in patients with an unstable long head of the biceps. These patients also may have rotator cuff symptoms. A trauma in which the subscapularis is torn may lead to the long head of the biceps being dislocated from the bicipital groove.

Physical Examination
Point tenderness of the biceps tendon, which is elicited within the bicipital groove, is a common finding. Speed's test,[50,51] Yergason's test,[52] and the biceps instability test[53] are used to identify long head of the biceps pathology. Biceps instability is identified by attempting to elicit a painful click while the arm is in full abduction and external rotation. Rupture of the long head of the biceps may be revealed by a dropped biceps deformity, which is identified by an indentation in the anterior shoulder and a lump on the anterolateral arm.

Imaging Studies
Standard shoulder radiographs are obtained to visualize any associated abnormalities. Ultrasound may be used to dynamically correlate sites of tenderness found on clinical examination with the involved pathology. The advantage of MRI is that it visualizes the biceps tendon in its groove, surrounding osteophytes, and any associated rotator cuff pathology.

Treatment
Reversible degeneration is expected when less than 25% of the overall tendon is involved, and the position of the tendon within the bicipital groove is normal; it is treated with observation of the biceps. Irreversible changes, including more than 25% partial-thickness tearing or fraying, tendon subluxation from the bicipital groove, or more than 25% reduction in tendon size, require surgical treatment.

Surgical treatment options include either biceps tenotomy or tenodesis.[54-58] Biceps tenodesis has potential advantages that include prevention of muscle atrophy, maintenance of elbow flexion and supination strength, avoidance of cramping pain, and avoidance of cosmetic deformity (A.A. Romeo, MD, unpublished data presented at American Society for Sports Medicine annual meeting, 2002). Tenodesis, therefore, is preferred for younger, more active, and thin patients. Open biceps tenodesis techniques have been well described,[41,57-59] and more recently, all-arthroscopic techniques have been advocated. Seikiya and associates[59] described a simple technique that sutures the biceps to the rotator interval. Gartsman and Hammerman[60] described an arthroscopic biceps tenodesis technique using suture anchors. Boileau and associates[61] reported a technique using interference screw fixation with the guide pin drilled through the humerus to tension the biceps within a bony tunnel. Klepps and associates[62] described a technique using interference screw fixation with tensioning of the biceps into a bony tunnel using suture anchors.

FIGURE 12

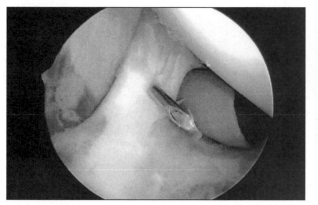

Percutanous spinal needle penetrates the biceps tendon.

FIGURE 13

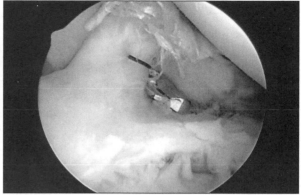

A monofilament suture is passed through the spinal needle and retrieved out the anterior portal.

Surgical Technique

The patient is placed in the lateral decubitus or beach chair position, and placement of the portals is marked on the patient's shoulder. After performance of standard diagnostic arthroscopy, an anterior working portal is fashioned just lateral to the coracoid process; a probe is used to pull the biceps tendon into the joint so that the part of the biceps that lies within the bicipital groove may be visualized. This step is required to avoid missing significant pathology (Figure 11). Tenodesis is then performed.

Percutaneous Intra-Articular Transtendon Technique (PITT)

This technique requires minimal instrumentation and fixes the biceps tendon to the rotator interval.[59] An 18-gauge spinal needle is passed percutaneously through the rotator interval tissue and through the biceps tendon (Figure 12). A No. 1 monofilament bioabsorbable suture is threaded through the needle and retrieved through the anterior cannula with a grasper, and the spinal needle is removed (Figure 13). A second spinal needle is passed similarly to pierce the biceps tendon next to the first suture. A second suture is threaded through the second needle and retrieved through the anterior cannula; then the spinal needle is removed. If desired, the monofiliament suture is exchanged for braided suture by tying the free ends of the monofilament to a braided suture and then shuttling the braided

FIGURE 14

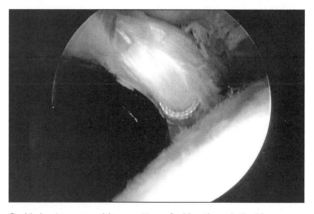

Braided suture passed in a mattress fashion through the biceps.

suture, creating a mattress stitch (Figure 14).

The steps are repeated to pass two to three sutures around the biceps tendon. The biceps tendon is then transected proximally, and the biceps origin attached to the glenoid is débrided with a motorized shaver (Figure 15). The camera is introduced in the subacromial space, and a lateral working portal is established. The sutures are located in the subacromial space and pulled through the lateral working portal. The sutures are tied using standard arthroscopic knot-tying techniques (Figure 16). If a rotator cuff tear is present, the proximal biceps may be incorporated into an anterior anchor used for fixation of the supraspinatous tear.

FIGURE 15

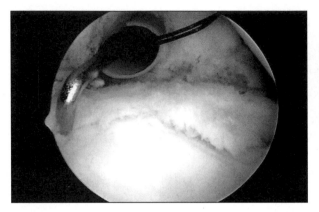

Tenotomy of the long head of the biceps has been performed and superior labrum débrided.

FIGURE 17

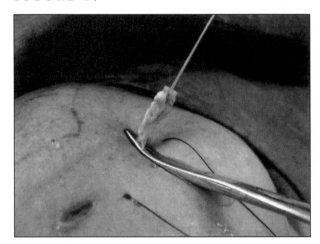

Biceps tendon delivered out of the anterior portal and whipstitch placed. *(Reproduced with permission form Ahmad CS, ElAttrache NS: Arthroscopic biceps tenodesis. Orthop Clin North Am 2003;34:499-506.)*

Interference Screw Fixation Technique

This technique fixes tendon to bone. As described in the PITT technique, sutures to control the biceps are percutaneously placed using a spinal needle passed through the proximal biceps (Figure 12). Monofilament sutures are placed through the needle and retrieved out the anterior portal (Figure 13). The biceps is then released from the superior labrum using an arthroscopic scissors or basket, and the residual stump is débrided to a stable, smooth margin (Figure 14).

FIGURE 16

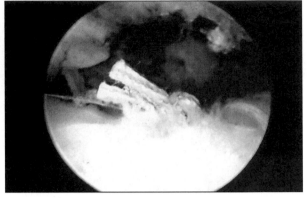

Suture is tied in the subacromial space for biceps tendon fixation.

The camera is moved from the intra-articular space to the subacromial space, and a lateral working portal is established just posterior and 2 cm lateral to the anterior edge of the acromion. A bursectomy is performed, followed by an acromioplasty, if necessary. After placement of the arthroscope into the lateral portal, the tendon is pulled out of the defect in the rotator cuff interval created by placement of the anterior cannula. After identification of the biceps sheath and the falciform ligament of the pectoralis major tendon, an arthroscopic blade or ablation device is used to transect them. The cannula is removed from the anterior portal, and the biceps tendon is brought out of the skin.

The shoulder and elbow are flexed and the humerus positioned in appropriate internal and external rotation to place the biceps directly under the anterior portal to maximize the length of tendon brought out of the skin. A 10- to 15-mm portion of the tendon may be excised to adjust its length to obtain proper tension for the bicipital groove tenodesis. The length of the intra-articular part of the biceps when the arm is adducted to the side has been estimated at 35 mm.[63] Because about 20 mm of tendon will be placed in a bone tunnel, the removal of an additional 10 to 15 mm will restore the appropriate length. A 20-mm whipstitch of No. 2 nonabsorbable suture is placed in the tendon to be introduced in the bone tunnel (Figure 17).

An accessory anterolateral portal is created 2 to 3 cm anterior to the anterolateral edge of the acromion. A shaver is used to débride soft tissue from the bicipital groove (Figure 18). After placement of a 2.4-mm guide

FIGURE 18

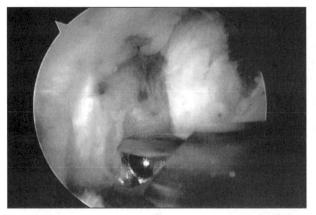

Biciptial groove débrided. *(Reproduced with permission form Ahmad CS, ElAttrache NS: Arthroscopic biceps tenodesis.* Orthop Clin North Am *2003;34:499-506.)*

FIGURE 19

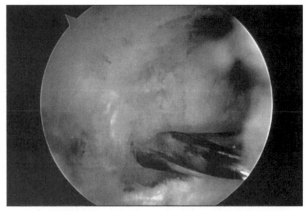

Guide pin placed in bicipital groove. *(Reproduced with permission form Ahmad CS, ElAttrache NS: Arthroscopic biceps tenodesis.* Orthop Clin North Am *2003;34:499-506.)*

FIGURE 20

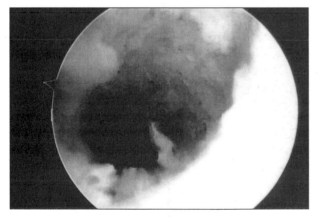

Bone tunnel created in bicipital groove. *(Reproduced with permission form Ahmad CS, ElAttrache NS: Arthroscopic biceps tenodesis.* Orthop Clin North Am *2003;34:499-506.)*

FIGURE 21

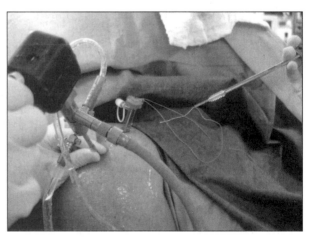

Interference screw on Bio-Tenodesis screwdriver with sutures being passed through the cannulation of the driver with a wire passer. Note camera position in lateral portal. *(Reproduced with permission form Ahmad CS, ElAttrache NS: Arthroscopic biceps tenodesis.* Orthop Clin North Am *2003;34:499-506.)*

pin in the center of the bicipital groove (Figure 19), a 25- to 30-mm deep bone tunnel is drilled (Figure 20). The cannula in the anterior portal is replaced with an 8.25-mm clear cannula in which the interference screw and driver are accommodated. An interference screw that is 1 mm smaller than the hole drilled is chosen and placed on the Arthrex Bio-Tenodesis screwdriver (Arthrex, Inc, Naples, FL). To control the biceps tendon, the whipstitch suture is passed through the screwdriver's cannula (Figure 21). The screwdriver and tendon are then inserted into the bone tunnel (Figure 22), and the screw is advanced over the tip of the screwdriver while constant tension is placed on the graft into the bone tunnel. Standard knot-tying techniques are used to tie the suture controlling the graft over the screw, thereby creating secondary fixation (Figure 23).

FIGURE 22

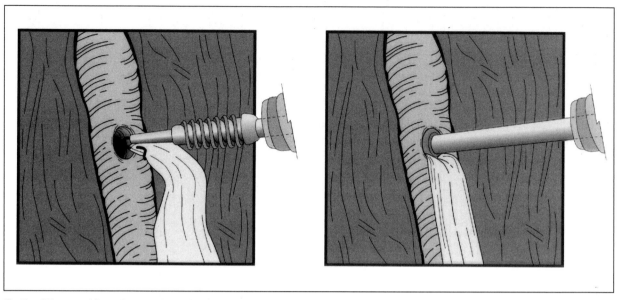

The tip of the screwdriver advances the graft into the tunnel and keeps constant tension on the graft while the screw is advanced. (*Reproduced with permission form Ahmad CS, ElAttrache NS: Arthroscopic biceps tenodesis.* Orthop Clin North Am *2003;34:499-506.*)

FIGURE 23

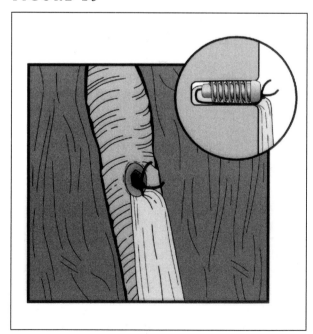

Fixation is achieved by both the interference screw and the sutures. (*Reproduced with permission form Ahmad CS, ElAttrache NS: Arthroscopic biceps tenodesis.* Orthop Clin North Am *2003;34:499-506.*)

Alternatively, open tenodesis may be performed through a mini-open deltoid-splitting approach to fix the biceps into the bicipital groove. A subpectoral inferior axillary approach also may be used. The incision is placed in the axilla, centered on the inferior border of the pectoralis major tendon. The biceps and coracobrachialis are identified, and the overlying fascia is incised longitudinally. A Hohmann retractor is placed under the pectoralis major to retract the muscle proximal and lateral. The long head of the biceps is brought out of the skin, and the length of the biceps required for appropriate tension is determined. At the location of the intended tenodesis, 25 mm is added to the biceps, and the remaining tendon is excised. Interference fixation of the biceps into the humerus is then obtained as described for the arthroscopic technique but with direct visualization.

Postoperative Protocol

Postoperative rehabilitation for patients undergoing combined rotator cuff repair and biceps tenodesis is focused on protection of the rotator cuff repair and restoration of motion. Active shoulder motion is started at 6 weeks, and it continues for 3 months, at which time resistive exercises begin. Patients undergoing isolated tenodesis immediately begin full passive and active-assisted shoulder motion exercises, but avoid active biceps flexion for 6 weeks. Full unlimited active elbow motion and resistive exercises are initiated at 6 weeks.

Outcomes

Excellent outcomes for open biceps tenodesis techniques have been reported.[41,54,55,57,58,64,65] A separate delto-pectoral incision is needed for the open techniques; this incision potentially increases postoperative pain and produces inferior cosmesis. Arthroscopic techniques aim to achieve adequate fixation strength with less morbidity. The more frequent performance of all-arthroscopic rotator cuff repairs favors a concomitant all-arthroscopic biceps tenodesis. Romeo (A.A. Romeo, MD, unpublished data presented at American Society for Sports Medicine annual meeting, 2002) reported comparison of open subpectoral and arthroscopic tenodesis techniques in a study that had 17 patients in each group and a follow-up of 7 months. No difference was found in American Shoulder and Elbow Society, Simple Shoulder Test, or Visual Analog Score testing. Both groups had a 6% rate of reoperation for persistent shoulder pain. Full comparison of the different techniques requires longer follow-up.

REFERENCES

1. Snyder SJ, Karzel RP, Del Pizzo W, Ferkel RD, Friedman MJ: SLAP lesions of the shoulder. *Arthroscopy* 1990; 6:274-279.
2. Davidson PA, Rivenburgh DW: Mobile superior glenoid labrum: A normal variant or pathologic condition? *Am J Sports Med* 2004;32:962-966.
3. Ide J, Maeda S, Takagi K: Normal variations of the glenohumeral ligament complex: An anatomic study for arthroscopic Bankart repair. *Arthroscopy* 2004;20:164-168.
4. Williams MM, Snyder SJ, Buford D Jr: The Buford complex: The "cord-like" middle glenohumeral ligament and absent anterosuperior labrum complex. A normal anatomic capsulolabral variant. *Arthroscopy* 1994;10:241-247.
5. Howell SM, Galinat BJ: The glenoid-labral socket: A constrained articular surface. *Clin Orthop Relat Res* 1989;243:122-125.

6. Soslowsky LJ, Flatow EL, Bigliani LU, Mow VC: Articular geometry of the glenohumeral joint. *Clin Orthop Relat Res* 1992;285:181-190.
7. Itoi E, Kuechle DK, Newman SR, Morrey BF, An KN: Stabilising function of the biceps in stable and unstable shoulders. *J Bone Joint Surg Br* 1993;75:546-550.
8. Rodosky MW, Harner CD, Fu FH: The role of the long head of the biceps muscle and superior glenoid labrum in anterior stability of the shoulder. *Am J Sports Med* 1994;22:121-130.
9. Burkart A, Debski RE, Musahl V, McMahon PJ: Glenohumeral translations are only partially restored after repair of a simulated type II superior labral lesion. *Am J Sports Med* 2003;31:56-63.
10. Levy AS, Kelly BT, Lintner SA, Osbahr DC, Speer KP: Function of the long head of the biceps at the shoulder: Electromyographic analysis. *J Shoulder Elbow Surg* 2001;10:250-255.
11. Yamaguchi K, Riew KD, Galatz LM, Syme JA, Neviaser RJ: Biceps activity during shoulder motion: An electromyographic analysis. *Clin Orthop Relat Res* 1997; 336:122-129.
12. Pagnani MJ, Deng XH, Warren RF, Torzilli PA, Altchek DW: Effect of lesions of the superior portion of the glenoid labrum on glenohumeral translation. *J Bone Joint Surg Am* 1995;77:1003-1010.
13. Bey MJ, Elders GJ, Huston LJ, Kuhn JE, Blasier RB, Soslowsky LJ: The mechanism of creation of superior labrum, anterior, and posterior lesions in a dynamic biomechanical model of the shoulder: The role of inferior subluxation. *J Shoulder Elbow Surg* 1998;7:397-401.
14. Clavert P, Bonnomet F, Kempf JF, Boutemy P, Braun M, Kahn JL: Contribution to the study of the pathogenesis of type II superior labrum anterior-posterior lesions: A cadaveric model of a fall on the outstretched hand. *J Shoulder Elbow Surg* 2004;13:45-50.
15. Kuhn JE, Lindholm SR, Huston LJ, Soslowsky LJ, Blasier RB: Failure of the biceps superior labral complex: A cadaveric biomechanical investigation comparing the late cocking and early deceleration positions of throwing. *Arthroscopy* 2003;19:373-379.
16. Morgan CD, Burkhart SS, Palmeri M, Gillespie M: Type II SLAP lesions: Three subtypes and their relationships to superior instability and rotator cuff tears. *Arthroscopy* 1998;14:553-565.
17. Kim TK, Queale WS, Cosgarea AJ, McFarland EG: Clinical features of the different types of SLAP lesions: An analysis of one hundred and thirty-nine cases. Superior labrum anterior posterior. *J Bone Joint Surg Am* 2003; 85-A:66-71.

18. Maffet MW, Gartsman GM, Moseley B: Superior labrum-biceps tendon complex lesions of the shoulder. *Am J Sports Med* 1995;23:93-98.

19. Field LD, Savoie FH III: Arthroscopic suture repair of superior labral detachment lesions of the shoulder. *Am J Sports Med* 1993;21:783-790.

20. Snyder SJ, Banas MP, Karzel RP: An analysis of 140 injuries to the superior glenoid labrum. *J Shoulder Elbow Surg* 1995;4:243-248.

21. Andrews JR, Carson WG Jr, McLeod WD: Glenoid labrum tears related to the long head of the biceps. *Am J Sports Med* 1985;13:337-341.

22. Burkhart SS, Morgan CD: The peel-back mechanism: Its role in producing and extending posterior type II SLAP lesions and its effect on SLAP repair rehabilitation. *Arthroscopy* 1998;14:637-640.

23. O'Brien SJ, Pagnani MJ, Fealy S, McGlynn SR, Wilson JB: The active compression test: A new and effective test for diagnosing labral tears and acromioclavicular joint abnormality. *Am J Sports Med* 1998;26:610-613.

24. Stetson WB, Templin K: The crank test, the O'Brien test, and routine magnetic resonance imaging scans in the diagnosis of labral tears. *Am J Sports Med* 2002;30:806-809.

25. Kim SH, Ha KI, Ahn JH, Choi HJ: Biceps load test II: A clinical test for SLAP lesions of the shoulder. *Arthroscopy* 2001;17:160-164.

26. Kibler WB: Specificity and sensitivity of the anterior slide test in throwing athletes with superior glenoid labral tears. *Arthroscopy* 1995;11:296-300.

27. Mimori K, Muneta T, Nakagawa T, Shinomiya K: A new pain provocation test for superior labral tears of the shoulder. *Am J Sports Med* 1999;27:137-142.

28. Guanche CA, Jones DC: Clinical testing for tears of the glenoid labrum. *Arthroscopy* 2003;19:517-523.

29. Bencardino JT, Beltran J, Rosenberg ZS, et al: Superior labrum anterior-posterior lesions: diagnosis with MR arthrography of the shoulder. *Radiology* 2000;214:267-271.

30. Mileski RA, Snyder SJ: Superior labral lesions in the shoulder: Pathoanatomy and surgical management. *J Am Acad Orthop Surg* 1998;6:121-131.

31. Cordasco FA, Steinmann S, Flatow EL, Bigliani LU: Arthroscopic treatment of glenoid labral tears. *Am J Sports Med* 1993;21:425-430.

32. Yoneda M, Hirooka A, Saito S, Yamamoto T, Ochi T, Shino K: Arthroscopic stapling for detached superior glenoid labrum. *J Bone Joint Surg Br* 1991;73:746-750.

33. Samani JE, Marston SB, Buss DD: Arthroscopic stabilization of type II SLAP lesions using an absorbable tack. *Arthroscopy* 2001;17:19-24.

34. Pagnani MJ, Speer KP, Altchek DW, Warren RF, Dines DM: Arthroscopic fixation of superior labral lesions using a biodegradable implant: A preliminary report. *Arthroscopy* 1995;11:194-198.

35. Segmuller HE, Hayes MG, Saies AD: Arthroscopic repair of glenolabral injuries with an absorbable fixation device. *J Shoulder Elbow Surg* 1997;6:383-392.

36. Burkart A, Imhoff AB, Roscher E: Foreign-body reaction to the bioabsorbable suretac device. *Arthroscopy* 2000;16:91-95.

37. Wilkerson JP, Zvijac JE, Uribe JW, Schurhoff MR, Green JB: Failure of polymerized lactic acid tacks in shoulder surgery. *J Shoulder Elbow Surg* 2003;12:117-121.

38. Kartus J, Kartus C, Brownlow H, Burrow G, Perko M: Repair of type-2 SLAP lesions using Corkscrew anchors: A preliminary report of the clinical results. *Knee Surg Sports Traumatol Arthrosc* 2004;12:229-234.

39. Kim SH, Ha KI, Kim YM: Arthroscopic revision Bankart repair: A prospective outcome study. *Arthroscopy* 2002;18:469-482.

40. Yian E, Wang C, Millett PJ, Warner JJ: Arthroscopic repair of SLAP lesions with a bioknotless suture anchor. *Arthroscopy* 2004;20:547-551.

41. Sethi N, Wright R, Yamaguchi K: Disorders of the long head of the biceps tendon. *J Shoulder Elbow Surg* 1999;8:644-654.

42. Burns WC II, Whipple TL: Anatomic relationships in the shoulder impingement syndrome. *Clin Orthop Relat Res* 1993;294:96-102.

43. Neer CS II: Anterior acromioplasty for the chronic impingement syndrome in the shoulder: A preliminary report. *J Bone Joint Surg Am* 1972;54:41-50.

44. Neer CS II: *Shoulder Reconstruction*. Philadelphia, PA, WB Saunders, 1990.

45. Neviaser TJ: The role of the biceps tendon in the impingement syndrome. *Orthop Clin North Am* 1987;18:383-386.

46. Burkhead WZ: The biceps tendon, in Rockwood CA, Matsen FAI (eds): *The Shoulder*. Philadelphia, PA, WB Saunders, 1990, pp 791-836.

47. Burkhead WZ: The biceps tendon, in Rockwood CAJ, Matsen FAI (eds): *The Shoulder*, ed 2. Philadelphia, PA, WB Saunders, 2000, pp 1009-1063.

48. Habermeyer P, Walch G: The biceps tendon and rotator cuff disease, in Burkhead WZ (ed): *Rotator Cuff Disorders*. Baltimore, MD, Williams and Wilkins, 1996, pp 142-59.

49. Slatis P, Aalto K: Medial dislocation of the tendon of the long head of the biceps brachii. *Acta Orthop Scand* 1979;50:73-77.

50. Neviaser RJ: Lesions of the biceps and tendinitis of the shoulder. *Orthop Clin North Am* 1980;11:343-348.

51. Gilcreest EL: Dislocation and elongation of the long head of the biceps brachii. An analysis of six cases. *Ann Surg* 1936;104:118-136.

52. Yergason RM: Supination sign. *J Bone Joint Surg* 1931;13:160.

53. Gerber C, Krushell RJ: Isolated rupture of the tendon of the subscapularis muscle. Clinical features in 16 cases. *J Bone Joint Surg Br* 1991;73:389-394.

54. Becker DA, Cofield RH: Tenodesis of the long head of the biceps brachii for chronic bicipital tendinitis. Long-term results. *J Bone Joint Surg Am* 1989;71:376-381.

55. Berlemann U, Bayley I: Tenodesis of the long head of biceps brachii in the painful shoulder: Improving results in the long term. *J Shoulder Elbow Surg* 1995;4:429-435.

56. Curtis AS, Snyder SJ: Evaluation and treatment of biceps tendon pathology. *Orthop Clin North Am* 1993;24:33-43.

57. Dines D, Warren RF, Inglis AE: Surgical treatment of lesions of the long head of the biceps. *Clin Orthop Relat Res* 1982;164:165-171.

58. Froimson AI: Keyhold tenodesis of biceps origin at the shoulder. *Clin Orthop Relat Res* 1975;112:245-249.

59. Sekiya LC, Elkousy HA, Rodosky MW: Arthroscopic biceps tenodesis using the percutaneous intra-articular transtendon technique. *Arthroscopy* 2003;19:1137-1141.

60. Gartsman GM, Hammerman SM: Arthroscopic biceps tenodesis: operative technique. *Arthroscopy* 2000;16:550-552.

61. Boileau P, Krishnan SG, Coste JS, Walch G: Arthroscopic biceps tenodesis: a new technique using bioabsorbable interference screw fixation. *Arthroscopy* 2002;18:1002-1012.

62. Klepps S, Hazrati Y, Flatow E: Arthroscopic biceps tenodesis. *Arthroscopy* 2002;18:1040-1045.

63. Mazzocca AD, Romeo AA: Arthroscopic biceps tenodesis in the beach chair position. *Oper Tech Sports Med* 2003;11:6-14.

64. Hichcock HH, Bechtol CO: Painful shoulder: Observations on role of tendon of long head of biceps brachii in its causation. *J Bone Joint Surg Am* 1948;30:263-273.

65. O'Donoghue DH: Subluxing biceps tendon in the athlete. *Clin Orthop Relat Res* 1982;164:26-29.

CHAPTER 5

ADHESIVE CAPSULITIS

CHARLES L. GETZ, MD
MATTHEW L. RAMSEY, MD
DAVID GLASER, MD
GERALD R. WILLIAMS, MD

Codman[1] coined the term frozen shoulder in 1934 and described it as a condition "difficult to define, difficult to treat, and difficult to explain from the point of view of pathology." Over 70 years later, most orthopaedic surgeons continue to reaffirm the difficulties faced when treating patients with this problem.

The term adhesive capsulitis was suggested as a more specific term than frozen shoulder by Neviaser[2] in 1945. The primary pathology in adhesive capsulitis, as opposed to other conditions that may be associated with loss of glenohumeral motion, is within the glenohumeral joint capsule—often in an otherwise normal shoulder. Zuckerman and Cuomo[3] have defined adhesive capsulitis as "a condition of uncertain etiology characterized by significant restriction of both active and passive shoulder motion that occurs in the absence of a known intrinsic shoulder disorder." Other conditions that can be associated with a frozen shoulder include glenohumeral arthritis, partial rotator cuff tears, fractures and malunions, and calcific tendinitis.

Shoulder stiffness is classified by its underlying etiology[4] (Table 1). Stiffness that develops following fracture or surgery is believed to be secondary to local inflammation and scarring. Intrinsic stiffness that develops suddenly occurs in patients who may have a systemic reason for the stiffness, such as diabetes mellitus, hyperthyroidism, or hypothyroidism. Despite other known causes that are directly or indirectly related to shoulder stiffness, most adhesive capsulitis develops without a known cause.

NATURAL HISTORY AND PATHOPHYSIOLOGY

Adhesive capsulitis is self-limiting in most patients. Its natural course is believed to include three phases: freezing, frozen, and thawing.[5] Phase I adhesive capsulitis is characterized by synovitis and painful motion (especially at the end range of motion), with little loss of motion, and it can be difficult to distinguish from subacromial pathology.[6] As the process continues, motion loss becomes more pronounced, with pain continuing and even increasing. The hallmark of phase II, or the frozen phase, is marked restriction of both active and passive range of motion. The pain in phase II disease is characteristically less severe than in phase I. In phase III, the stiffness progressively resolves. The time frame for a patient to recover from adhesive capsulitis can be 2 to 3 years.[7] Although most patients are functional, performing daily activities with little or tolerable pain, residual loss of motion, and activity- or weather-related pain are common.[7-9]

The exact mechanism of the local and humeral inflammatory factors that cause adhesive capsulitis is not understood. An inflammatory response is the end result of a complex interplay of the immune system.[10,11] Bulgen and associates[10,12] found a significant decrease in the immunoglobulin A blood levels that persisted after recovery from adhesive capsulitis. They also found a decreased lymphocytic response in patients with adhesive capsulitis compared with unaffected controls. Perhaps most intriguing was a finding of impaired cell-mediated immunity and an increase in immune

TABLE 1

Classification of Shoulder Stiffness

Adhesive capsulitis
    Idiopathic
Associated with systemic process
    Diabetes mellitus
    Hyperthyroidism
    Hypothyroidism
Posttraumatic
    Fracture malunion
    Postfracture union
    Minor trauma
    Postsurgical

complex levels in patients with adhesive capsulitis compared with unaffected controls. A relationship to HLA-B27 has been suggested,[10,12] but to date evidence supporting this theory is conflicting.

Although the exact molecular basis for adhesive capsulitis is unknown, the histologic changes are well defined. Changes within the synovium include an inflammatory response, perivascular infiltration, capsular thickening, and fibrosis.[2] Neviaser[6] used arthroscopy to identify four specific stages: stage 1 consists of a mild erythematous synovitis; stage 2 consists of acute synovitis with adhesion in the dependent folds; stage 3 is characterized by maturation of adhesions with less synovitis; and stage 4 consists of chronic adhesions without synovitis.

The rotator interval has been proposed by several authors as a major contributor in the development of adhesive capsulitis. DePalma[13] reported autopsy findings of contracted rotator intervals and thickening of the capsule and rotator cuff. Ozaki and associates[14] and Neer and associates[15] independently observed contracture of the rotator interval and its effects on restricting shoulder motion. Although Neer and associates also emphasized that no one structure was responsible for the development of adhesive capsulitis, they hypothesized that when the rotator interval (including the biceps tendon and coracohumeral ligament) become inflamed and thickened, the structures are transformed to increase glenohumeral contact pressures.

Endocrine disorders, such as diabetes mellitus, hypothyroidism, hypoadrenalism, triglyceridemia, and corticotropin deficiency, have been associated with adhe-

sive capsulitis.[16] In general, when adhesive capsulitis occurs in patients with diabetes mellitus, it is more severe, more prolonged, and less responsive to treatment. The incidence of bilaterality is also higher in patients with diabetes mellitus. Although it has not been reported, we have noticed a correlation between adhesive capsulitis and the presence of family members with diabetes mellitus and hypothyroidism, even if the patient does not have either of these conditions. It seems rare that a patient in our practice with adhesive capsulitis has neither diabetes mellitus nor hypothyroidism or does not have a blood relative with one of these two conditions.

Trauma about the shoulder girdle has long been recognized as a source of stiffness, either from prolonged immobilization or from inciting capsular inflammation. In addition to stiffness from fracture malunion, fracture nonunion, and hardware prominence, minor traumatic events often start an inflammatory process within the shoulder that leads to stiffness.

EVALUATION

History and physical examination findings will vary according to the stage of the disease; however, pain is the most common presenting symptom. Because severe pain is most characteristic of the freezing or synovitic phase, most patients present in phase I. Patients between ages 40 and 60 years are affected most commonly, and women are affected more often than men.[17] A history of minor trauma, such as lifting a bag of groceries or reaching into the back seat of the car, is not uncommon. However, most often, no traumatic inciting event can be identified. Rarely, more substantial trauma, such as fractures, surgery, dislocations, falls, and car accidents, may be elucidated. A personal history of diabetes or thyroid disorders should raise the index of suspicion for adhesive capsulitis.

In the early stages of adhesive capsulitis, before substantial loss of passive motion has occurred, the diagnosis can be difficult. The shoulder may be acutely painful, as in many other shoulder conditions. In this scenario, adhesive capsulitis easily can be mistaken for primary rotator cuff disease. Unfortunately, most of the commonly prescribed treatments for rotator cuff disease, especially surgery, may exacerbate the signs and symptoms of adhesive capsulitis. Therefore, the clinician should have a high index of suspicion for adhesive capsulitis in all patients with the spontaneous onset of shoulder pain, especially if they have diabetes mellitus or hypothyroidism or have a blood relative with either of these two conditions.

Although distinguishing between primary rotator cuff disease and adhesive capsulitis can be difficult, several physical findings are suggestive of adhesive capsulitis. The hallmark of adhesive capsulitis is simultaneous loss of both active and passive range of motion. The degree of motion loss required to distinguish between adhesive capsulitis and primary rotator cuff disease associated with posterior capsular contracture, for example, has not been quantified. The active and passive range of motion must be determined.

To assess elevation, the patient is asked to elevate the affected arm. If a lack of terminal elevation exists, the examiner's hand is placed under the patient's elbow to determine the degree to which passive motion exists in this plane. Active and passive range of motion should be compared with ranges in the unaffected extremity. Similarly, the patient's active external range of motion with the arms at the sides is compared with the patient's passive range of motion. Although few data exist with regard to the amount of passive motion loss required to make a diagnosis of adhesive capsulitis, 20% loss compared with the normal side should at least alert the clinician to the possibility of the condition. The presence of a lag sign, external rotation weakness, or pain with resisted external rotation suggests a pathologic source related to the rotator cuff.

Capsular irritation signs can help distinguish early adhesive capsulitis from primary rotator cuff disease. With the arm at the patient's side, the anterior capsule can be stretched by gently externally rotating the arm past the point where passive motion would normally end. The presence of synovitis or capsular irritation, which is characteristic of adhesive capsulitis, will cause this maneuver to be painful. This reaction is in contradistinction to primary impingement-related rotator cuff disease, which is more painful with resisted active external rotation within the physiologic range of motion. This distinction between painful passive stretch of the anterior capsule and painful resisted active external rotation may help the clinician distinguish between adhesive capsulitis and primary rotator cuff disease or impingement, respectively.

A similar maneuver to assess irritation of the inferior capsule can be performed with the arm abducted to 90° in the plane of the scapula. The examiner supports the patient's elbow in this position and externally rotates the arm past the point where passive external rotation usually would end. The pain generated by this maneuver can be compared with the pain generated by internal rotation with the arm abducted and forward flexed (Hawkins manuever).[18] If the pain generated by stretching the inferior capsule is substantially greater than that generated by the Hawkins manuever, a diagnosis of adhesive capsulitis, as opposed to primary rotator cuff disease or impingement, is supported. Other tests that support a diagnosis of adhesive capsulitis include biceps provocative tests such as Speed's[19] or Yergason's[20] and resisted internal rotation with the subscapularis on slight stretch.

The diagnosis of adhesive capsulitis is relatively straightforward when substantial loss of active and passive motion is present. However, in the early stages of the disease, the diagnosis may be more difficult. Although none of the above tests are specific or pathognomonic for adhesive capsulitis, the totality of all the findings, combined with experience, a high index of suspicion, and good history taking, will allow the examiner to arrive at the correct diagnosis. The importance of subsequent reexamination(s) to help clarify the diagnosis should not be underestimated.

Radiographic Studies

Plain radiographs are required to effectively evaluate the painful and/or stiff shoulder. Idiopathic adhesive capsulitis and glenohumeral arthritis have similar clinical pictures. Therefore, plain radiographs are helpful to exclude a diagnosis of arthritis. In patients with posttraumatic or postsurgical stiffness, radiographs can reveal prominent hardware, nonunion, malunion, missed dislocations, heterotopic ossification, or glenohumeral arthritis. Bone quality also should be noted on the plain radiographs if manipulation is to be considered.

Advanced imaging studies rarely are required for the diagnosis of idiopathic adhesive capsulitis but may have a role in posttraumatic or postsurgical stiffness.[21] The integrity of a rotator cuff repair, for example, can be determined in a patient who developed stiffness after the repair by obtaining an MRI scan. Similarly, CT may be needed to evaluate hardware location in a patient after open reduction and internal fixation. MRI also may be useful to help elucidate a cause for continued pain in a patient whose stiffness has resolved.

TREATMENT

Nonsurgical Treatment

When treating patients with adhesive capsulitis, the clinician should remember that 85% of patients recover most of their shoulder function and experience substantial pain relief with no treatment at all.[7] This recovery may take 2 years or more; therefore, patients with adhesive capsulitis should be encouraged to be patient. Given this natural history, the mainstay of treatment of idiopathic adhesive capsulitis has been nonsurgical, consisting of some combination of physical therapy, nonsteroidal anti-inflammatory drugs, short-term oral steroids, analgesics, and intra-articular corticosteroid injections. Fortunately, most patients will improve with these modalities. The failure rate of nonsurgical treatment is approximately 10% if patients are followed for 1 to 3 years.[7]

The benign nature of adhesive capsulitis has been challenged by several authors. Clarke and associates[22] found 42% of patients with motion restriction at 6 years follow-up. Shaffer and associates[8] also reported a more bleak outcome for patients with adhesive capsulitis, with 56% still having restricted motion at nearly 10 years follow-up. Despite physical findings of restricted motion, most patients perceive minimal loss of function.[7]

Patients who fail to respond to these nonsurgical treatments may be candidates for surgery. Patients with adhesive capsulitis who fail nonsurgical treatment fall into one of two categories: nonresponders and surrenderers. Nonresponders have complied with nonsurgical management for an extended period of time (eg, 1 to 1.5 years), and their shoulders remain stiff and/or painful. Surrenderers realize that they may improve if they allow an extended period of time to pass; however, they are no longer willing or able to tolerate the pain and functional restrictions. In our surgical practice, surrenderers substantially outnumber nonresponders. However, every attempt should be made to continue nonsurgical management in both categories of failure as long as a documented improvement in range of motion is occurring. This period usually is at least 6 to 12 months.

Many reports have confirmed that manipulation is an effective treatment. However, critics of the procedure cite reports of humerus fractures and brachial plexus injuries. Some surgeons suggest that gaining internal rotation by manipulation alone is also difficult.[23]

Patients with posttraumatic and postsurgical stiffness also can be treated nonsurgically. However, they are less likely to respond than patients with idiopathic adhesive capsulitis. Neither posttraumatic nor postsurgical stiffness is believed to be self-limiting. Therefore, surgical intervention is indicated after a shorter period of nonsurgical treatment than in idiopathic adhesive capsulitis.

Arthroscopy and Adhesive Capsulitis

The role of arthroscopy has changed extensively over the past 25 years. The arthroscope initially was used to help identify the synovial and capsular processes that occur as adhesive capsulitis progresses. As noted earlier, Neviaser[6] identified four stages of the appearance of adhesive capsulitis. At about the same time, the arthroscope was further investigated as a means to produce capsular distention. Brisement or capsular distention had been used before arthroscopy with some success.[24-26] With the arthroscope, the pressure of the joint could be measured and the capsule distended during diagnostic arthroscopy.[27] Arthroscopic brisement had similar success.

Manipulation traditionally has been the definitive treatment of recalcitrant adhesive capsulitis. The arthroscope was used initially by surgeons to identify the structures that were disrupted during manipulation, and it also was used as an adjunct to manipulation. The disrupted structures were identified as the anterior and inferior capsule.

Once the structures that were disrupted during manipulation were identified, the principle of sectioning the affected areas of the capsule was applied to develop anterior arthroscopic capsular release.[28] Limited anterior sectioning of the capsule in patients whose capsules were not disrupted by manipulation yielded encouraging results.[29,30] Patients were improved but some lacked internal rotation.[23] A posterior capsular release in addition to the anterior arthroscopic release was studied and found to be beneficial in improving internal rotation.[4,31-34] Arthroscopic capsular release also has been found to be an effective means of improving motion in patients with posttraumatic and postsurgical stiffness.[4,32]

Authors' Technique

The choice of anesthetic is ultimately up to the patient after a discussion with the anesthesiologist. However, an interscalene block can be very helpful with postoperative pain control. Because pain often is a problem in patients with adhesive capsulitis, some consideration should be given to an interscalene block, even if the patient prefers a general anesthetic.

Although the role of manipulation before arthroscopy is debated because of the potential risk of fracture from forceful manipulation, I prefer gentle manipulation before insertion of the arthroscope. After induction of anesthesia, a gentle manipulation is performed with the patient placed in the supine position. The surgeon stands on the same side of the table as the affected shoulder, places one hand on the superior aspect of the shoulder as the other grasps the middle of the humerus, and moves the arm into elevation in the scapular plane. The motion should be smooth, with a gradual increase of the force applied. As capsular tearing occurs, the surgeon will feel and hear a pop, which will be followed by an increase in the range of motion.

Following manipulation in the scapular plane, the arm is placed in 90° of abduction and externally rotated, and the humerus is extended slightly posterior to the scapular plane. The humerus is then moved into internal rotation at 90° of elevation in the scapular plane, followed by cross-body adduction at 90° of elevation. Finally, the arm is brought to the side and the humerus is rotated externally. If passive range of motion after manipulation equals that of the asymptomatic side in all planes, no arthroscopic procedure is performed. If limitations of motion remain, arthroscopic capsular release is indicated.

To perform arthroscopic capsular release, the patient is placed into a beach chair position, and the affected shoulder is prepared and draped for surgery. A 4.5-mm arthroscope is placed in the shoulder through a standard posterior portal (Figure 1). When sufficient blood has been lavaged from the joint to permit visualization, an anterior portal is established using an outside-in technique. The portal should be centered horizontally between the humerus and the glenoid and vertically between the upper border of the subscapularis and the biceps tendon.

Any material that is obscuring the view can be removed with a shaver. Hyperemic synovium may bleed when shaved; therefore, electrocautery should be available. Once visualization has been established, attention is turned to the rotator interval and the superior portion of the capsule (Figure 2). An arthroscopic electrocautery is placed through the anterior portal, and the

FIGURE 1

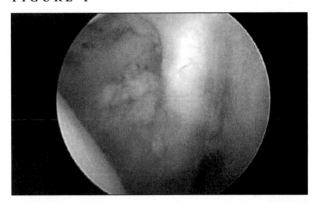

On visualization of the joint with the arthroscope, the capsule is often hyperemic and thickened.

FIGURE 2

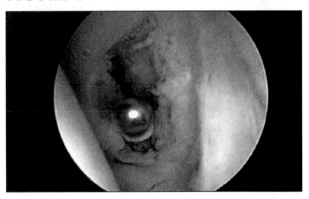

Electrocautery can perform much of the release while limiting bleeding from the hypervascular tissue.

superior glenohumeral ligament, rotator interval, and coracohumeral ligament are divided by incising the rotator interval tissue superior to the subscapularis and continuing superiorly to the anterior border of the supraspinatus muscle. This boundary is approximated by the anterior extent of the biceps anchor. The rotator interval tissue can be quite thickened. Incision is complete when the posterior aspect of the conjoined tendon can be visualized. The electrocautery is then brought superior to the biceps tendon, and the superior capsule is incised, starting at the anterior border of the supraspinatus and continuing as far posterior as possible. The capsular incision should be directly superior to the biceps anchor and superior labrum and should be stopped when the supraspinatus muscle fibers can be visualized through the capsulotomy.

The middle glenohumeral ligament can be very hypertrophic in patients with adhesive capsulitis; therefore, the electrocautery is used to transect it. This ligament is seen best by externally rotating the arm 15° or 20°, and it should be distinguished from the subscapularis tendon to prevent injury to the latter structure. The electrocautery can then be used to divide the upper portion of the inferior glenohumeral ligament (anterior band). The interval between the subscapularis muscle fibers and the inferior glenohumeral ligament is identified best when release of the anterior band occurs adjacent to the labrum. A blunt-tipped punch then can be passed in this interval to dissect the subscapularis away from the capsule, and the capsulotomy can be continued inferiorly with the punch. In most instances, the capsular rent that occurred during manipulation will be visualized as the anteroinferior margin of the glenoid is reached.

If the manipulation did not produce a capsular rent, the arthroscope is maneuvered into the remaining axillary recess, and the lens is rotated into a superior orientation. This maneuver not only visualizes the remaining capsule, but also places the capsule under tension to aid dissection. An up-biting, blunt-tipped punch is used to bluntly develop the plane between the capsule and the overlying, more superficial soft tissues—primarily the subscapularis muscle belly. The capsulotomy is then continued to the 6 o'clock position. If the punch cannot be placed outside the capsule in a closed position to create a space before the capsulotomy is performed, the capsulotomy should not be performed because of potential danger to the axillary nerve.

At this point, the arthroscopic instruments should be removed and the patient's range of motion should be reassessed to see whether the releases have returned it. If lack of internal rotation still exists, the arthroscope is placed into the anterior portal, and an arthroscopic electrocautery is placed into the posterior portal. The previously performed superior capsulotomy is continued posteriorly and inferiorly, taking care to stay close (1 cm) to the glenoid margin. At the posteroinferior glenoid margin, the branch of the axillary nerve to the teres minor is at risk; therefore, a blunt-tipped punch can be passed outside the capsule to dissect away any adjacent structure before performing the capsulotomy. Again, the inferior capsular rent caused by the manipulation usually can be visualized as the posteroinferior portion of the glenoid is approached.

Following completion of the release, the arm is manipulated gently through a range of motion to ensure all adhesions are broken and full motion is restored. Often, a small bridge of capsule will remain following capsular release. This bridge is broken during the final manipulation. The affected arm is placed into a sling. While the patient is still under regional anesthesia and awake, the patient's arm may be brought through a range of motion so that the patient is aware that normal motion has been restored and is possible.

Postoperative Care

The gains made during the procedure will be lost if the patient does not begin physical therapy shortly after surgery. In revision situations, we admit the patient for therapy, and we recommend an in-dwelling scalene catheter during the hospital stay. In primary situations, we have been successful in discharging patients who previously arranged to begin supervised passive range-of-motion exercises the following morning. This plan must be discussed with the patient before surgery so that all arrangements can be made before the patient comes to the hospital for surgery. The patient is questioned in the holding area before surgery and, if physical therapy has not been set up, the surgery is cancelled.

Some surgeons have reported strapping the patient's arm to the stretcher or bed in an elevated position, presumably to reinforce to the patient the fact that full elevation is now possible. We have not found this procedure to be necessary and are concerned about placing a patient into an extreme glenohumeral position after the patient has had all static glenohumeral stabilizers transected and proprioception anesthetically blocked.

Patients undergoing arthroscopic capsular release must be ready to commit a substantial amount of time and energy in the first 3 months following surgery. Gains made in range of motion may be maintained if the patient is able to begin physical therapy either the day of surgery or 1 day postoperatively. The first 6 weeks of exercises focus on range of motion. If a selective capsular release or manipulation has been performed, then the routine is tailored to increase the motion that was lost before the procedure.

Range-of-motion exercises include an overhead pulley, passive forward flexion in the supine position, passive external rotation in the supine position, passive external rotation with the arm abducted to 90°, cross-body adduction, internal rotation with the hand behind the back, and internal rotation with the arm at 90° (Figure 3).

Postoperative visits are scheduled at 1 to 2 weeks to determine patient compliance and that the proper program is being performed. In addition, the sutures are removed, and the wounds are inspected for infection. Early use of nonsteroidal anti-inflammatory drugs may be helpful to reduce overall narcotic consumption and to decrease postrehabilitation inflammation. If, at the first postoperative visit, external rotation with the arm at the side is less than 30°, consideration is given to an intra-articular corticosteroid injection. A call to the physical therapist may also be warranted to be explicit about what is expected.

At 6 weeks postoperatively, range of motion should be 70% to 80% of that of the unaffected side.

If pain at the ends of motion is diminishing, more aggressive passive stretching may be instituted. However, strengthening exercises should not be added until passive stretch at the end of motion is pain free or nearly pain free, which usually takes at least 3 months. Adding strengthening exercises before this time may result in increased pain, decreased ability to tolerate passive mobilization, and regression of range of motion. Most patients who have undergone a capsular release for adhesive capsulitis will regain their strength spontaneously when the motion returns and the pain subsides. Therefore, we rarely emphasize strengthening during any portion of the rehabilitation.

Complete recovery often takes a full year. However, if the return of motion is complete in the operating room, the rehabilitation protocol is appropriate, and the patient is compliant, the patient will be off pain medication and able to perform daily activities at 3 to 4 months postoperatively.

Results

Results of studies that have examined the efficacy of arthroscopic capsular release have been positive. In 1979, Conti[35] described a procedure in which he used a trochar to divide the rotator interval, manipulated the shoulder, and placed corticosteroid into the joint. Improvement in 16 of 18 patients was noted by 3 weeks, and the other two patients improved by 6 months.

Pollock and associates[29] reported the results of 30 patients who failed to regain external rotation motion after manipulation under anesthesia. These patients underwent immediate arthroscopic débridement of the coracohumeral ligament and anterosuperior capsule. No attempt was made to release the inferior capsule. At an average follow-up of 31 months, 50% of the patients were graded excellent, and 33% were graded satisfactory. There was a 17% unsatisfactory rate overall, with a higher failure rate in patients with diabetes.

In a 1995 prospective study, Ogilvie-Harris and associates[36] compared 20 patients who underwent manipulation with 20 patients who underwent arthroscopic capsular release. Their arthroscopic technique consisted of four steps: (1) removal of synovium within the rotator interval, (2) division of the anterosuperior glenohumeral ligament and anterior capsule, (3) partial division of the subscapularis tendon, but not muscle, and (4) division of the inferior capsule. Patients in both groups benefited from the intervention, and there was a strong trend toward better motion in the patients who underwent release, but significance was not reached. However, a significant number of patients who underwent release returned to normal motion (17 of 20) compared with the manipulation group (9 of 20).

Segmuller and associates[23] reported the results of 24 patients (26 shoulders) who underwent anterior capsular release and anterior synovectomy followed by manipulation. Overall, 88% of the patients were satisfied with the procedure. Range of motion was within 20% of normal for 77% of the patients for forward flexion, 82% of the patients for external rotation, and only 50% of the patients for internal rotation. The lack of gains in internal rotation led to interest in adding a capsulotomy of the posterior capsule.

Warner and associates[32] discussed the surgical technique of a posterior capsular release in a series of patients with postsurgical contracture. The addition of the posterior release did not add any complications and aided in restoring internal rotation.

In a separate report, Warner and associates[28] proposed a step-wise manipulation and anterior release in patients with refractory idiopathic adhesive capsulitis. No attempts were made to release the posterior or inferior capsule because the authors believed that manipulation could break the restrictive elements once the anterior structures were divided. The results of 23 patients at an average follow-up of 39 months were reported. As a group, the range of motion improvement was significant in all planes. No significant difference was detected between

FIGURE 3

Occupational & Physical Therapy Department
University of Pennsylvania Health System

Shoulder Phase I ROM Exercises

These exercises are intended to increase your range of motion. Move the shoulder to the position where slight discomfort is felt. In time (may be days) you should be able to move further into the range with less pain. Occasionally, you may need to push the shoulder into a more painful position but never force the motion. You should not experience pain for greater than 1-2 hours after exercising. You may use moist heat for 10-20 minutes before stretching and use ice for 10-20 minutes after exercise.

Hold for _____ seconds, do _____ times, _____ times a day.

Elevation

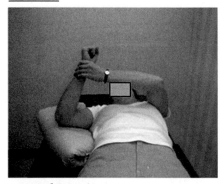 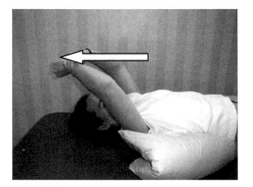

External Rotation

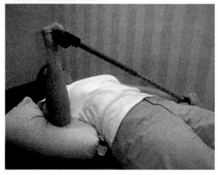

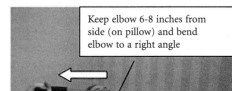

Keep elbow 6-8 inches from side (on pillow) and bend elbow to a right angle

Keep hand below waist

Limit rotation to _____ degrees

Active Assisted Elevation

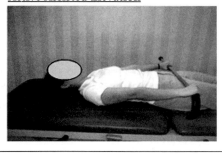 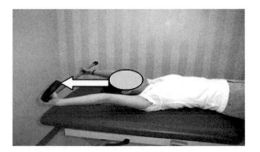

FIGURE 3 (CONT.)

Occupational & Physical Therapy Department
University of Pennsylvania Health System
Shoulder Phase II ROM Exercises

These exercises are intended to increase your range of motion. Move the shoulder to the position where slight discomfort is felt. In time you should be able to move further into the range with less pain. Occasionally, you may need to push the shoulder into a more painful position but never force the motion. You should not experience significant pain for greater than 1-2 hours after exercising. You may use moist heat for 10-20 minutes before stretching and use ice for 10-15 minutes after exercise.

Extension

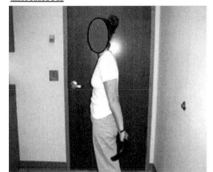

Hold for _____ seconds, do _____ times, _____ times a day.

Horizontal Adduction

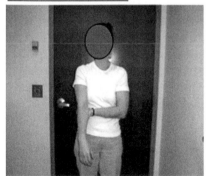
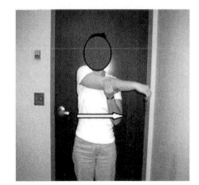

Hold for _____ seconds, do _____ times, _____ times a day.

Internal Rotation

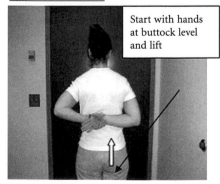
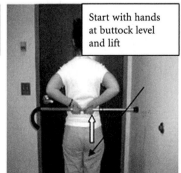

Start with hands at buttock level and lift

Start with hands at buttock level and lift

Do one of these internal rotation exercises.

Hold for _____ seconds, do _____ times, _____ times a day.

Handouts used to teach patients a home stretching program. *(Courtesy of Martin Kelly, PT, and Brian Leggin, PT.)* ROM, range of motion.

postoperative forward flexion of the affected and unaffected sides, but a small significant difference was noted in internal and external rotation range of motion.

Harryman and associates[33] reported the results of 30 patients who underwent a more extensive capsular release that included the posterior and inferior capsule when necessary. Significant functional improvement in all parameters at an average of 33 months was reported. Other authors have reported high rates of success with a more extensive 360° capsular release.[4,31,34]

As mentioned previously, arthroscopy has been used to treat postsurgical contracture. In Warner and associates'[32] report of 11 patients at 27-month follow-up, range of motion had been increased significantly in all planes, and the mean Constant and Murley score[37] improved 43 points. Holloway and associates[4] reported a series in which the results of postsurgical stiffness, postfracture stiffness (the fracture was not malunited), and idiopathic adhesive capsulitis were studied. All groups showed an improvement in motion, functional scores, and pain scores. However, the patients with postsurgical stiffness had a significantly lower final functional score, pain score, and satisfaction score.

Berghs and associates[38] reported results in 25 patients who underwent arthroscopic capsular release and manipulation for idiopathic adhesive capsulitis without concomitant procedures. The results supported earlier studies and showed a diminished outcome in patients with diabetes.

The durability of the procdure recently has been shown by Ide and Takagi.[39] In their report of 42 patients with a mean follow-up of 7.5 years, 84% of the patients had excellent outcomes, 7% had good outcomes, and 9% were poor. One third of the patients underwent arthroscopic acromioplasty at the same time.

Complications

Despite the technical difficulty of arthroscopic capsular release, there have been relatively few reports of complications. Recurrent stiffness or failure to regain motion has been the most common failure of both release and manipulation and has been discussed previously. Concerns about injury to the axillary nerve have been published, but only one transient nerve palsy has been reported.[33] The rate of axillary nerve injuries is unknown but seems to be low.

Another concern is of possible chondral injury from introduction of the trochar into the contracted joint. The combination of a thickened capsule that requires increased force to penetrate, a decreased capsular space to slip into the joint safely, and a decreased ability of the humeral head to translate and avoid the trochar combine to make initial introduction of the arthroscope more difficult than during arthroscopy of a supple joint. Manipulation of the shoulder before introduction of the arthroscope should allow easier introduction and decrease risk. If the surgeon remains concerned, insufflation of the joint with sterile saline may be beneficial.

Immediate postoperative dislocation has been reported by Harryman and associates.[33] However, the patient did not develop any recurrent instability, and recurrent instability has not been reported as a complication after release. To avoid immediate dislocation, we do not strap the patient's arm overhead. An attempt is made to move the patient's arm while the block is still in effect to demonstrate that motion has been regained.

IMPLICATIONS FOR THE FUTURE

The use of arthroscopy in conjunction with manipulation for recalcitrant adhesive capsulitis should decrease the force required to regain motion. The use of gentler manipulation hopefully will decrease the risk of fractures and brachial plexus injuries. Arthrosocpy also gives the treating physician a chance to assess the shoulder for other sources of pathology that may be contributing to the patient's pain.

As orthopaedic surgeons become more aware of the morbidity of adhesive capsulitis, they will be tempted to shorten the period of nonsurgical treatment and proceed to manipulation and release. Although this temptation should be resisted, it is questionable how long a patient with no motion, substantial pain, and a good surgical solution reasonably can be asked to persist with marginally successful nonsurgical management. Certainly, further studies are required to determine the usefulness of arthroscopic capsular release in the early stages of adhesive capsulitis. Adequate data currently exist to support the use of arthroscopic capsular release in patients with recalcitrant adhesive capsulitis.

REFERENCES

1. Codman EA: *The Shoulder*. Boston, MA, Thomas Todd, 1934.

2. Neviaser JS: Adhesive capsulitis of the shoulder: Study of pathological findings in periarthritis of the shoulder. *J Bone Joint Surg Am* 1945;27:211-222.

3. Zuckerman JD, Cuomo F: Frozen shoulder, in Matsen FA III, Fu FH, Hawkins RJ (eds): *The Shoulder: A Balance of Mobility and Stability*. Rosemont, IL, Americn Academy of Orthopaedic Surgeons, 1993, pp 253-267.

4. Holloway GB, Schenk T, Williams GR, Ramsey ML, Iannotti JP: Arthroscopic capsular release for the treatment of refractory postoperative or post-fracture shoulder stiffness. *J Bone Joint Surg Am* 2001;83:1682-1687.

5. Harryman DT II: Shoulders: Frozen and stiff. *Instr Course Lect* 1993;42:247-257.

6. Neviaser TJ: Adhesive capsulitis. *Orthop Clin North Am* 1987;18:439-443.

7. Reeves B: The natural history of the frozen shoulder syndrome. *Scand J Rheumatol* 1975;4:193-196.

8. Shaffer B, Tibone JE, Kerlan RK: Frozen shoulder: A long-term follow-up. *J Bone Joint Surg Am* 1992;74:738-746.

9. Binder AI, Bulgen DY, Hazleman BL, Roberts S: Frozen shoulder: A long-term prospective study. *Ann Rheum Dis* 1984;43:361 364.

10. Bulgen DY, Hazleman BL: Immunoglobulin-A, HLA-B27, and frozen shoulder. *Lancet* 1981;2:760.

11. Bulgen D, Hazleman B, Ward M, McCallum M: Immunological studies in frozen shoulder. *Ann Rheum Dis* 1978;37:135-138.

12. Bulgen DY, Hazleman BL, Voak D: HLA-B27 and frozen shoulder. *Lancet* 1976;1:1042-1044.

13. DePalma AF: Loss of scapulohumeral motion (frozen shoulder). *Ann Surg* 1952;135:193-204.

14. Ozaki J, Nakagawa Y, Sakurai G, Tamai S: Recalcitrant chronic adhesive capsulitis of the shoulder: Role of contracture of the coracohumeral ligament and rotator interval in pathogenesis and treatment. *J Bone Joint Surg Am* 1989;71:1511-1515.

15. Neer CS II, Satterlee CC, Dalsey RM, Flatow EL: The anatomy and potential effects of contracture of the coracohumeral ligament. *Clin Orthop Relat Res* 1992;280:182-185.

16. Bunker TD, Esler CN: Frozen shoulder and lipids. *J Bone Joint Surg Br* 1995;77:684-686.

17. Baslund B, Thomsen BS, Jensen EM: Frozen shoulder: Current concepts. *Scand J Rheumatol* 1990;19:321-325.

18. Hawkins R, Abrams JS: Impingement syndrome in the absence of rotator cuff tear (stages 1 and 2). *Orthop Clin North Am* 1987;18:373-382.

19. Neviaser RJ: Lesions of the biceps and tendonitis of the shoulder. *Orthop Clin North Am* 1980;11:343-348.

20. Yergason R: Supination sign. *J Bone Joint Surg Am* 1931;13:160.

21. Sher JS, Iannotti JP, Williams GR, et al: The effect of shoulder magnetic resonance imaging on clinical decision making. *J Shoulder Elbow Surg* 1998;7:205-209.

22. Clarke G, Willis LA, Fish WW, Nichols PJ: Preliminary studies in measuring range of motion in normal and painful stiff shoulders. *Rheumatol Rehabil* 1975;14:39-46.

23. Segmuller HE, Taylor DE, Hogan CS, Saies AD, Hayes MG: Arthroscopic treatment of adhesive capsulitis. *J Shoulder Elbow Surg* 1995;4:403-408.

24. Gilula LA, Schoenecker PL, Murphy WA: Shoulder arthrography as a treatment modality. *AJR Am J Roentgenol* 1978;131:1047-1048.

25. Fareed DO, Gallivan WR Jr: Office management of frozen shoulder syndrome: Treatment with hydraulic distension under local anesthesia. *Clin Orthop Relat Res* 1989;242:177-183.

26. Andren L, Lundberg BJ: Treatment of rigid shoulders by joint distension during arthrography. *Acta Orthop Scand* 1965;36:45-53.

27. Hsu SY, Chan KM: Arthroscopic distention in the management of frozen shoulder. *Int Orthop* 1991;15:79-83.

28. Warner JJ, Allen A, Marks PH, Wong P: Arthroscopic release for chronic, refractory adhesive capsulitis of the shoulder. *J Bone Joint Surg Am* 1996;78:1808-1816.

29. Pollock RG, Duralde XA, Flatow EL, Bigliani LU: The use of arthroscopy in the treatment of resistant frozen shoulder. *Clin Orthop Relat Res* 1994;304:30-36.

30. Andersen NH, Sojbjerg JO, Johannsen HV, Sneppen O: Frozen shoulder: Arthroscopy and manipulation under general anesthesia and early passive motion. *J Shoulder Elbow Surg* 1998;7:218-222.

31. Watson L, Dalziel R, Story I: Frozen shoulder: A 12-month clinical outcome trial. *J Shoulder Elbow Surg* 2000;9:16-22.

32. Warner JJ, Allen AA, Marks PH, Wong P: Arthroscopic release of postoperative capsular contracture of the shoulder. *J Bone Joint Surg Am* 1997;79:1151-1158.

33. Harryman DT II, Matsen FA III, Sidles JA: Arthroscopic management of refractory shoulder stiffness. *Arthroscopy* 1997;13:133-147.

34. Nicholson GP: Arthroscopic capsular release for stiff shoulders: Effect of etiology on outcomes. *Arthroscopy* 2003;19:40-49.

35. Conti V: Arthroscopy in rehabilitation. *Orthop Clin North Am* 1979;10:709-711.

36. Ogilvie-Harris DJ, Biggs DJ, Fitsialos DP, MacKay M: The resistant frozen shoulder: Manipulation versus arthroscopic release. *Clin Orthop Relat Res* 1995;319:238-248.

37. Constant CR, Murley AH: A clinical method of functional assessment of the shoulder. *Clin Orthop Relat Res* 1987;214:160-164.

38. Berghs BM, Sole-Molins X, Bunker TD: Arthroscopic release of adhesive capsulitis. *J Shoulder Elbow Surg* 2004;13:180-185.

39. Ide J, Takagi K: Early and long-term results of arthroscopic treatment for shoulder stiffness. *J Shoulder Elbow Surg* 2004;13:174-179.

CHAPTER 6

GLENOHUMERAL AND ACROMIOCLAVICULAR JOINT ARTHRITIS

LOUIS U. BIGLIANI, MD
SEAN BAK, MD

Application of shoulder arthroscopy has grown significantly in the past 2 decades. Routine shoulder arthroscopy allows both glenohumeral evaluation and access to the acromioclavicular (AC) joint. Arthroscopic treatment of glenohumeral arthritis has not been as extensively investigated as that of knee arthritis, but successful pain relief in many series has been documented.[1-3] Benefits of arthroscopy in shoulder arthritis extend beyond simple débridement of the glenohumeral joint because additional intra-articular and bursal pathology often accompanies arthritis.[3,4] The definitive treatment of AC arthritis is distal clavicle resection, and, since its introduction in the 1980s, the success of the arthroscopic version of this procedure has equaled and, in some studies, surpassed the success of the open approach.[5-10]

GLENOHUMERAL ARTHRITIS

The most reliable means of restoring function and eliminating pain in patients with glenohumeral arthritis has been shoulder replacement arthroplasty since its inception by Neer[11] in 1974. Despite the continuing improvement in shoulder replacement arthroplasty, some patients are not ideal candidates for this procedure. Concerns about the durability of prosthetic joints in young patients or those with relatively early arthritis are legitimate, and the postponement of arthroplasty may be prudent. At the other end of the age spectrum are older patients with symptomatic arthritis for whom glenohumeral arthroplasty may be contraindicated because of medical fragility. Deltoid dysfunction or inability to comply with postarthroplasty rehabilitation and limitations preclude shoulder arthroplasty regardless of the severity of the arthritis. Arthroscopy may be a reasonable alternative for such patients, given the clear understanding that relief often is both incomplete and temporary (S.C. Weber, J.I. Kauffman, unpublished data presented at the American Shoulder and Elbow Society annual meeting, 2004).

Arthroscopic treatment of osteoarthritic joints recently has been the focus of intense scrutiny. Much of this scrutiny has been centered on knee arthroscopy and the value of débridement in the presence of advanced arthritis.[12-14] A key difference between the arthritic knee and the arthritic shoulder is the high prevalence of coexistent subacromial pathology in glenohumeral arthritis.[3,15] A crucial factor common to the success of arthroscopy for arthritis of the shoulder or the knee is patient selection. It generally is accepted that débridement of end-stage osteoarthritis (OA) is not indicated, whereas arthroscopy remains a viable option for patients with clear mechanical symptoms and early-stage OA.[16]

Evaluation

Evaluation of the patient with glenohumeral arthritis begins with a complete history. Hand dominance and symptoms affecting the contralateral shoulder are determined. The patient's occupational and recreational activities should be defined. The onset and quality of the pain also should be determined. Arthritic pain generally is insidious in onset, and acute onset of pain, especially if associated with minor trauma, may be indicative of other pathology such as a rotator cuff or proximal biceps tear. Systemic symptoms indicative of an inflammatory arthropathy or infection should be elicited.

Previous treatment must be documented. Most patients with arthritis will experience at least temporary relief with nonsteroidal anti-inflammatory drugs (NSAIDs). Previous use of steroids or alcohol or the presence of other risk factors for osteonecrosis should be explored. Any history of shoulder surgery should raise suspicion of postcapsulorrhaphy or thermal arthropathy.

Perhaps the most critical aspect of the history in a patient with arthritis who is being considered for arthroscopy is a very clear description of the patient's current limitations and postoperative expectations for pain and function. In the younger patient, motion restriction can be restored reliably by means of arthroscopic release, assuming the patient has the commitment to comply with the arduous postoperative regimen. When pain is the main symptom, the patient must clearly understand that relief is unlikely to be complete and will be of an unpredictably temporary duration.

Physical Examination

The patient is examined while disrobed to the waist. Scars may indicate previous surgery such as an instability repair. The examiner should look for any asymmetry or muscular atrophy from both anterior and posterior.

Range-of-motion (ROM) assessment is instrumental in planning capsular releases in those patients in whom stiffness is a major component of the pathology. The classic natural history of glenohumeral arthritis is an initial loss of external rotation followed by varying degrees of stiffness in other planes. Internal rotation contracture may be quite pronounced after capsulorrhaphy. Forward elevation, external rotation (with the arm at the side and with the arm abducted 90°), internal rotation, and cross-body adduction are recorded. Comparison with the contralateral side is mandatory. Subtle changes in ROM are often more evident with the patient supine.

Crepitus with motion is a common symptom and physical finding in arthritis, and it typically occurs with

---

TABLE 1

Kellgren/Lawrence Radiographic Grading of Osteoarthritis

Grade 0	Normal
Grade 1	Minute osteophytes
Grade 2	Osteophytes; joint space preserved
Grade 3	Moderate joint space narrowing
Grade 4	Joint space narrowing, subchondral sclerosis

---

rotation in the glenohumeral joint, although it often does not occur until a relatively advanced stage. The compression-rotation test described by Ellman and associates[15] is useful because it causes pain in the patient with early, mild arthritis. Posterior joint-line tenderness frequently is noted.

Signs of concomitant pathology, such as impingement, AC arthritis, and biceps pain, must be identified to offer the patient the best chance at postoperative relief. Integrity of the rotator cuff should be assessed, although it rarely is compromised in the patient with OA.[17] Significant rotator cuff deficits are common in rheumatoid arthritis (RA). Selective injection of the glenohumeral joint, subacromial space, and AC joint can help define the source of pain.

Radiographic Evaluation

A complete shoulder series comprises five views, including true AP views of the shoulder with the humerus in internal rotation, external rotation, and neutral, an axillary lateral view, and a supraspinatus outlet view. The axillary lateral view is necessary to gauge version of the glenoid and position of the head on the glenoid; the supraspinatus outlet view is used to evaluate acromial morphology. The radiographic findings in OA are graded as to severity based on the Kellgren and Lawrence (K/L) system[18] (Table 1 and Figure 1). Without the enhancement of weight bearing, the true degree of OA in the upper extremity, especially in the early stages, can be underestimated.[4,19] RA usually is associated with symmetric joint space narrowing, osteopenia, and subchondral erosions and, with advanced disease, medialization

FIGURE 1

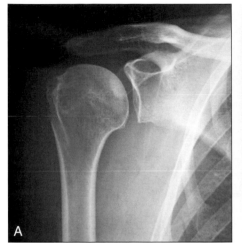
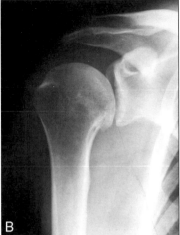
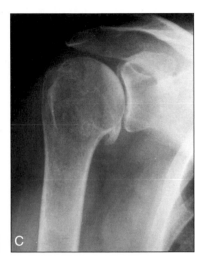

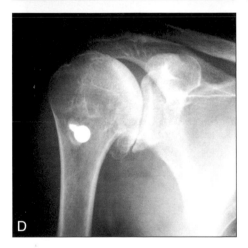

Examples of the four grades of osteoarthritis after Kellgren and Lawrence. **A,** Grade 1. **B,** Grade 2. **C,** Grade 3. **D,** Grade 4.

of the glenoid. Patients with a history of instability repair, especially a Bristow or Latarjet procedure, or patients who have a significant decrease in external rotation (less than 30°), often will have eccentrically posterior wear of the glenoid.[20] MRI and CT, although not typically pursued for isolated OA, frequently are already available or may be obtained to evaluate coexistent processes.

Indications

Osteoarthritis

Idiopathic OA is characterized by pathologic changes in the chondrocytes and extracellular matrix of articular cartilage, resulting in its progressive deterioration. Although OA often is depicted as resulting from wear and tear, the degree to which the wear and tear actually contributes to the degenerative process remains unclear.[21] The degradation of articular cartilage in OA begins with increasing permeability of the extracellular matrix to water. This permeability theoretically renders the matrix more susceptible to production of proteases, most notably matrix metalloproteinase (MMP), by chondrocytes that also are initiated in this stage. This production is followed by a chondrocyte response to matrix injury with a combination of both proliferative repair factors and degradative enzymes. A delicate balance between these opposing factors may persist for

TABLE 2	
Outerbridge Classification	
Modified Outerbridge Grade	**Appearance**
I	Softening/blistering
II	Fissuring/fibrillation
III	Deep ulceration
IV	Exposed subchondral bone

FIGURE 2

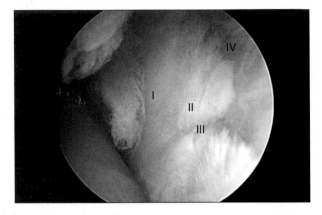

Arthroscopic view of the left glenohumeral joint from the posterior portal. Appearance of glenohumeral osteoarthritis with typical posterior wear pattern. Various zones of chondromalacia labeled according to the modified Outerbridge classification.

FIGURE 3

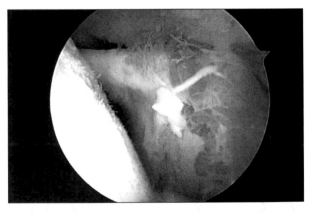

Arthroscopic view of the left shoulder from the posterior viewing portal showing marked synovitis in the posterosuperior glenohumeral joint.

years. The final stage occurs as this balance finally shifts in favor of MMP activators, and chondrocyte death accelerates. Development of osteophytes parallels articular changes and becomes more prominent as the disease progresses. In the late stages of OA, osteophytes may become tender and often tether the joint capsule contributing to loss of motion.[22-25]

Arthroscopy has proved to be an important diagnostic tool in glenohumeral OA. As the use of shoulder arthroscopy for indications other than arthritis has risen, so has the incidental discovery of significant preradiographic glenohumeral arthritis. It is during these early, radiographically subtle stages of OA that the efficacy of arthroscopic débridement is maximized. Chondral defects are graded according to a modification of the original Outerbridge classification[26] (Table 2 and Figure 2).

Arthroscopic treatment of OA is, in its simplest form, a joint lavage. This procedure, on the molecular level, aims to clear the joint of catabolic enzymes and growth factors that mediate the degradation of articular cartilage. On a slightly larger scale, loose bodies and tiny cartilage particles that cause mechanical and synovial irritation, respectively, are removed.[27] Neither the extent to which the lavage fluid is able to penetrate and remove destructive enzymes nor how long it takes for the inevitable reaccumulation is known. The benefit of lavage is supported indirectly by evidence that introduction of matrix breakdown products into the synovial fluid can stimulate further degradation of the matrix.[28] Therefore, it follows that removal of these molecules may impair degradation.

Débridement of the joint is conducted concurrently with the lavage. Although synovitis is not the major component of idiopathic OA, most affected joints do exhibit some degree of secondary synovial inflamma-tion, the relatively easy débridement of which may contribute to pain relief (Figure 3). The degree of relief obtained from chondroplasty is unclear, although it is more likely to be therapeutic in the presence of large unstable flaps of cartilage because they suggest a mechanical component of irritation. Treatment of articular cartilage defects is an area of intense investigation, and arthroscopic techniques involving microfracture and abrasion arthroplasty have been successful in several studies.[29-32] Loose bodies have the ability to generate painful mechanical episodes, and their removal

FIGURE 4

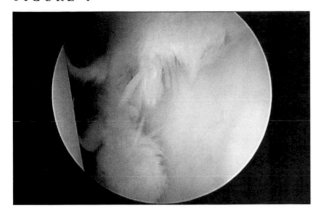

Arthroscopic view of the left shoulder from the posterior viewing portal. Typical quality of labral fraying in osteoarthritic shoulder.

usually is helpful. Removal of small osteophytes may have a minor role in pain relief and restoration of motion by releasing their mechanical tethering effect. Large osteophytes usually are indicative of advanced disease for which arthroscopic treatment is contraindicated.

Concomitant pathology is rather common and also can be addressed via shoulder arthroscopy.[3,15] The osteoarthritic shoulder typically exhibits a significant degree of stiffness for which capsular release can result in substantial functional gain. Indications for capsular release in the arthritic shoulder have been set at a 15° to 20° deficit in any plane as compared with the contralateral shoulder.[1] Biceps tendon inflammation can be treated with arthroscopic release of the long head of the biceps with or without tenodesis. Labral fraying is common in the arthritic shoulder and was likened to degenerative meniscal tears of the knee by Ogilvie-Harris (Figure 4). Débridement of these lesions yielded favorable results in his series.[2] Although labral fraying is frequently present, unstable SLAP lesions are not common. We recommend simple débridement of labral pathology with biceps tenodesis rather than labral repair in the presence of a type II or IV SLAP lesion. Literature on the treatment of unstable SLAP lesions in the arthritic patient is scant, but in our experience, the repair of labral detachment in these patients may result in decreased range of motion postoperatively. Subacromial bursitis is a common finding (as high as 92% in one series) during arthroscopy of the arthritic shoulder.[3] Rotator cuff tears can be addressed by débridement of partial-thick-

TABLE 3

Potential Benefits of Arthroscopic Treatment of an Arthritic Glenohumeral Joint

Joint lavage and removal/dilution of degradative enzymes
Débridement of inflamed synovium
Improvement of joint mechanics by removal of loose bodies, cartilage flaps, and release of capsular contractures
Treatment of subacromial bursitis and other concomitant pathology
Diagnosis/prognosis

TABLE 4

Indications for Arthroscopic Treatment of Glenohumeral Arthritis

Failed nonsurgical treatment
Concentric joint
K/L radiographic grade 1 to 2
Minimal deformity

ness tears or repair of full-thickness tears.

Ultimately, progression of OA cannot be prevented by any current treatment short of arthroplasty, but arthroscopic débridement in the early stages can alleviate symptoms and may slow progression. Arthroscopy of the glenohumeral joint can be beneficial for K/L grade 1 to 2 disease that has failed nonsurgical management.[2,3] Chondral lesions in excess of 2 cm^2 indicate a poor prognosis for long-term pain relief.[1] Given the high rate of associated subacromial pathology and favorable results after bursectomy, inspection of the subacromial space is an essential component of the arthroscopy. Arthroscopic débridement in grade 3 disease without eccentric wear may be considered, depending on individual factors such as age and medical comorbidities that may preclude arthroplasty in that particular patient's foreseeable future. Radiographic grade 4 correlates with the third stage of OA at which point the balance has tipped far in favor of degradation of hyaline cartilage, and the use of arthroscopy is minimal. Benefits of arthroscopic débridement of the arthritic shoulder are summarized in Table 3 with indications listed in Table 4.

TABLE 5

Mayo Clinic Classification of RA Radiographic Appearance

Mayo Clinic Stage	Radiographic Appearance
I	Normal to mild osteoporosis
II	Narrowing of joint, architecture remains intact
IIIA	Joint erosion (moderate)
IIIB	Joint erosion (severe)
IV	Gross destruction of joint

FIGURE 5

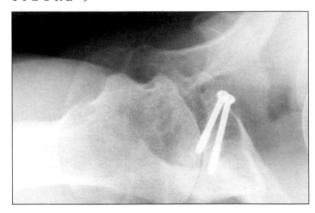

Axillary radiograph of the shoulder with characteristic posterior wear after anterior stabilization procedure.

Inflammatory Arthritis

RA affects a younger patient population than OA; however, good results have been reported for glenohumeral arthroplasty in this population, partially because of their overall less active lifestyle.[33,34] Although a completely different disease process than OA, RA also is a product of an intricate inflammatory cascade that ultimately results in joint destruction. Thus, simple glenohumeral débridement may offer some benefit similar to that seen in OA. Early stages of the disease are characterized by pain and stiffness with proliferation of a thickened synovium and primary involvement of the soft tissues with sparing of the joint. During this stage, synovectomy can result in dramatic pain relief if the joint architecture has remained relatively normal.[35,36] Complete synovectomy can be done arthroscopically without taking down any major muscle group around the glenohumeral joint, thus speeding return of motion and overall recovery. This technique also is useful in patients with pigmented villonodular synovitis and synovial chondromatosis, the latter of which benefits significantly from removal of the multiple loose bodies.

The Mayo Clinic classification of RA radiographic stages was originally described for the elbow but can be applied to the glenohumeral joint[37] (Table 5). Arthroplasty generally is indicated for stages III and greater involvement; while arthroscopy, joint débridement, and synovectomy can be considered for stages I and II disease refractory to nonsurgical management. Unlike OA, rotator cuff tears and a reactive subacromial bursitis are relatively common in the shoulder with RA, and both can be addressed at the time of arthroscopy.[38]

Postcapsulorrhaphy

Postcapsulorrhaphy arthritis is a well-recognized consequence of nonanatomic stabilization procedures for anterior glenohumeral instability. Modern stabilization techniques have significantly minimized this problem, although it still is observed when overtightening of the anterior structures occurs.[17,39] The glenohumeral joint with postcapsulorrhaphy arthritis typically will have asymmetric posterior wear and is quite tight anteriorly, with significant lack of external rotation (Figure 5). Arthroscopy of the joint is indicated when concentricity is reasonably well-maintained and degenerative changes are limited to stage I or II. Perhaps the principal benefit of arthroscopy in patients with glenohumeral arthritis is capsular release for restoration of external rotation, which not only improves function but may impede development of further arthritis. Instability after such release is not observed routinely.[39]

Osteonecrosis and Thermal Arthropathy

Osteonecrosis of the humeral head often affects a younger patient population than primary OA. Etiology varies but the natural history is pain followed by progressive joint destruction, the end stage of which is best treated with replacement arthroplasty. Thermal arthropathy or chondrolysis after a thermal arthroscopic procedure has been reported recently by multiple authors.[40-42]

The value of arthroscopy in these patients lies primarily in the débridement and removal of loose bodies and

FIGURE 6

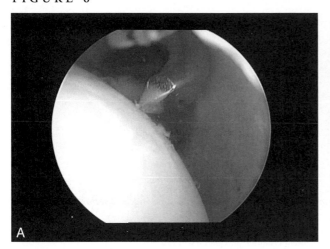 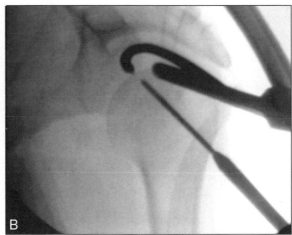

A, Arthroscopic view of the left shoulder from the posterior viewing portal. The anterior cruciate ligament targeting guide is in good position at the center of the humeral head. **B,** Fluoroscopic view of a well placed pin just prior to drilling for core decompression of the humeral head.

unstable flaps of articular cartilage from the joint. In the case of thermal arthropathy, the degree of chondrolysis may not be evident on plain radiographs, and arthroscopy may be necessary for diagnosis. Arthroscopically assisted core decompression of the humeral head has been reported, with the proposed advantage of more accurate determination of the extent of osteonecrosis. This procedure also uses an anterior cruciate ligament tunnel guide, which, when combined with the direct visualization of arthroscopy, can prevent articular penetration of the drill[42] (Figure 6).

Technique

Anesthesia and Positioning

Beach chair versus lateral positioning and method of anesthesia are matters of individual surgeon preference. We perform arthroscopy with the patient in the beach chair position using interscalene regional anesthetic. Motion and stability always are examined under anesthesia, with particular attention paid before capsular release to confirm that true mechanical restriction exists as opposed to guarding, which can be quite convincing in some patients during the office examination. Use of a bed that has a cutaway section at the level of the shoulder and also is equipped with a pneumatic arm positioner has proved helpful during arthroscopy. Complete access to the shoulder is necessary because arthritic pathology typ-

ically involves the joint in global fashion, requiring viewing from both anterior and posterior portals.

Débridement

The arthroscope is introduced from a standard posterior portal, and diagnostic arthroscopy is performed. Traction, applied with the pneumatic arm holder or by an assistant and accompanied by gentle introduction of the arthroscope above the humeral head, can prevent damage to the articular surface in these narrow, relatively nondistensible joints. The anterior portal is established in outside-in fashion just lateral to the coracoid process, coming into the rotator interval. The biceps tendon is visualized, and a probe is used to pull it medially into the joint, allowing visualization of most of its sheathed portion. We have a low threshold for tenodesis when there is evidence of fraying or inflammation because biceps tendinitis can be a major contributor to shoulder pain in the patient with arthritis. The labrum often is frayed, and it is débrided with a motorized shaver.

Articular surfaces are probed with an instrument of known width, allowing for accurate quantification of cartilage lesions. Unstable flaps are débrided judiciously with the shaver, whereas removal of stable areas of cartilage is avoided. Thorough and systematic examination of the joint is necessary to identify any loose bodies, many of which are purely cartilaginous and, therefore,

FIGURE 7

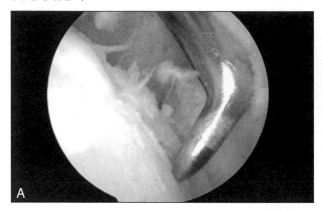
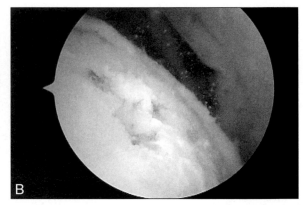

Arthroscopic view of the left shoulder from the posterior viewing portal. **A,** Chondral pick positioned perpendicular to an articular defect of the humeral head. **B,** View of three puncture holes in the humeral head after microfracture with exposure of subchondral bone.

are not evident on plain radiographs. The axillary pouch and the subscapularis recess are two common sites where these fragments may be found. Viewing from the anterior portal with an accessory anterior instrument portal often is necessary for extraction of loose bodies from the subscapularis recess.

Synovectomy

The synovitis of idiopathic OA is usually a secondary response to the joint destruction that begins in the articular cartilage itself. Débridement of involved areas yields a varying degree of pain relief. In contrast, the synovitis of inflammatory arthritis and chondromatosis is the primary source of joint pathology, and complete synovectomy is necessary not only for pain relief, but also to minimize the chance of recurrence. Therefore, both viewing and working from anterior and posterior portals is necessary, often with the creation of multiple accessory portals. Removing all synovium while maintaining integrity of the capsule and rotator cuff can be challenging at times; however, every effort must be made to avoid violation of the capsule because multiple areas of capsular damage may lead to scarring and subsequent contracture. Extensive synovectomy generally is last in the series of intra-articular procedures because it often produces bleeding. However, some degree of initial synovectomy is invariably necessary in the inflamed joint to permit adequate visualization.

Capsular Release

Details of capsular release are outlined elsewhere in this monograph. The classic loss of external rotation is addressed with an anterior capsular release. Lack of internal rotation is addressed with a posterior release, although this is only occasionally necessary in the patient with arthritis and is contraindicated if there is any evidence of posterior wear or subluxation.

Abrasion Chondroplasty and Microfracture

Discrete, contained, full-thickness cartilage lesions in younger patients are amenable to abrasion chondroplasty and microfracture. Additional options include autologous cartilage implantation and osteochondral autograft transfer, which currently are performed via glenohumeral arthrotomy. Chondral picks of varied angles are available for microfracture, which is necessary for perpendicular orientation with respect to the lesion. This microfracture is relatively straightforward for humeral head lesions because rotation of the head facilitates placement, but it may be necessary to create several accessory portals for treatment of glenoid lesions to allow proper placement of multiple puncture sites in the subchondral bone (Figure 7). Abrasion arthroplasty is performed gently with a burr. The creation of divots or craters in the subchondral bone is discouraged because one of the goals for this procedure is a congruent surface that must be maintained if the procedure is to be successful. The goal of these two theoretically similar procedures is the creation of bleeding and subsequent clot in the subchondral bone, allowing for accumulation of growth factors and mesenchymal cells that ultimately may lead to replacement of the lesion with fibrocartilage.

Concomitant Pathology

Subacromial bursitis and AC joint arthritis frequently accompany glenohumeral arthritis and can be distinguished with selective injections. These also can be addressed during the same arthroscopy and are described elsewhere in this chapter. Rotator cuff tears are rather uncommon in the presence of glenohumeral arthritis, but they also may be managed arthroscopically.

Postoperative Course

The primary goal in the treatment of arthritic joints is restoration of joint function, an integral component of which is motion. When capsular release is performed, the patient is admitted overnight with an indwelling catheter that remains in place through the first therapy session. Otherwise, arthroscopy is typically an outpatient procedure, and we encourage motion as soon as comfortable. In the absence of rotator cuff repair, the affected arm is placed in a sling for several days, after which both passive and active-assisted physical therapy is initiated. Return to standard daily activities occurs at 4 to 6 weeks.

Results

Literature on the topic of arthroscopic treatment of glenohumeral arthritis is sparse. Published results are predominantly favorable, although most results are relatively short-term. Early reports helped shape indications for this procedure and, clearly, patient selection and mild arthritic changes are the keys to success.

Ogilvie-Harris and Wiley[2] reported the results of arthroscopic débridement for OA in 54 patients in 1986. At 3-year follow-up, results were successful in two thirds of the patients with mild degeneration but in only one third of the patients with severe degenerative disease. Best results were seen in patients with preoperative stiffness that was released at the time of débridement or in patients with labral fraying that was débrided during the arthroscopy.

The coexistence of subacromial pathology is clearly detailed in the literature. Ellman and associates[15]

reported on a series of patients who had shoulder arthroscopy for presumed impingement and were found to have significant full-thickness chondral defects of the humeral head and, to a lesser degree, the glenoid. In addition to glenohumeral débridement, 15 of 18 patients received subacromial decompressions; results were positive but no long-term follow-up was available. Weinstein and associates[3] reported on a series of 25 patients who underwent arthroscopic débridement of the glenohumeral joint with concomitant subacromial bursectomy. Follow-up averaged 34 months, and 80% of the patients exhibited good to excellent results. Favorable results correlated with early-stage arthritis, and the authors concluded that arthroscopy of the arthritic glenohumeral joint was indicated for early arthritis in which the joint space and congruence were preserved.

The extent of articular damage recently has been shown to bear prognostic implications. Cameron and associates[1] reviewed results of glenohumeral débridement of patients with known grade IV osteochondral lesions and achieved an overall satisfaction rate of 88%. Failure of the procedure was associated with lesions larger than 2 cm^2.

Although sustained relief has been seen in multiple studies, the progression of arthritis essentially is not altered by arthroscopic débridement. Thirty-five patients with a minimum of 2-year follow-up after arthroscopic débridement for glenohumeral osteoarthritis were recently presented (S.C. Weber, J.I. Kauffman, unpublished data presented at the American Shoulder and Elbow Society annual meeting, 2004). Substantial pain relief was observed in most patients at the 3-month mark; however, only 28% reported a good result at long-term follow-up. Survivorship was 85% at 5 years using glenohumeral arthroplasty as the end point, but all patients exhibited radiographic progression of the disease.

Complications

Complications after glenohumeral and/or subacromial arthroscopy are infrequent.[3] In arthroscopic capsular release, axillary nerve injury is rare. Potential complications are those inherent to shoulder arthroscopy itself, including fluid extravasation and temporary postoperative drainage, instrument breakage, infection, and iatrogenic articular injury. Although arthroplasty is clearly the gold standard in treatment of glenohumeral arthritis, arthroscopy provides a low morbidity option with the potential for significant improvement in the carefully selected patient.

Future Directions

Current indications for arthroscopic treatment of the arthritic shoulder require a concentric joint. The typical wear pattern of OA is posterior glenoid erosion. O'Driscoll[43] recently explored glenoidplasty, which, in addition to a standard débridement, involves a contouring of the glenoid back to a more concentric surface via an arthroscopic approach. Preliminary results indicate some success in short-term pain relief, although longer follow-up of this novel approach will be necessary before expanding the indications of arthroscopy to more advanced stages of glenohumeral arthritis.

Successful glenohumeral arthrodesis using arthroscopic assistance and percutaneous fixation has been reported.[44] Thorough débridement of articular cartilage is performed arthroscopically with the goal of creating congruent surfaces of subchondral bone on the humeral and glenoid sides. Direct arthroscopic visualization is used to augment fluoroscopic placement of hardware.

ACROMIOCLAVICULAR JOINT ARTHRITIS

The AC joint is a diarthrodial synovial joint that, despite its small surface area, is responsible for linkage of the upper extremity to the thorax and, thus, is responsible for transmission of considerable force. It is supported superiorly by the AC ligaments that stabilize in the anteroposterior direction and by the thick coracoclavicular ligaments that prevent excessive craniocaudal displacement.[45] As a result of the scapulothoracic articulation, minimal motion occurs at the AC joint.[46] Idiopathic OA is the most common form seen in the AC joint, although the joint also is susceptible to inflammatory and posttraumatic forms of arthritis. AC joint arthritis often coexists with subacromial impingement and rotator cuff disease, and, thus, arthroscopic treatment of this arthritis has been refined significantly since the introduction of shoulder and subacromial arthroscopy.[47,48] Although missed AC joint arthritis remains a leading cause of failed anterior subacromial decompression, treatment based on radiographs alone may lead to overdiagnosis. Posttraumatic arthritis also occurs with injury to the AC joint and frequently is accompanied by some incongruence, typically in the superoinferior plane. Distal clavicular osteolysis occurs in patients, primarily men, in their third or fourth decade and is highly associated with heavy weight training involving motions in the forward flexed and overhead positions.[49]

Evaluation

History and Physical Examination

Patients with AC joint arthritis often give a history consistent with impingement and rotator cuff tendinitis because the three often coexist. These patients will have characteristic pain with motion below the shoulder level; forward flexion is not painful in isolated AC joint arthritis, although patients with concomitant impingement will have pain in the overhead range. Classic patients are heavy laborers and weight lifters, and AC joint arthritis commonly is seen in the older overhead athlete. Pain while fastening a brassiere or reaching in the back pocket with the affected arm often is described. Night pain and pain while lying on the affected shoulder are common symptoms. Trauma involving the AC joint certainly can predispose patients to degenerative changes, and the clinician must take care to identify any instability because AC joint separations of grade II and higher have an unacceptably high failure rate with distal clavicle resection alone.[6,50] Typically, the pain of primary AC joint arthritis is gradual in onset and atraumatic.

Examination usually reveals tenderness over the often quite prominent AC joint. Pain in the vicinity of the AC joint and, frequently, crepitus with passive cross-body adduction or extension and internal rotation of the shoulder (eg, reaching in the back pocket) are the most reliable physical findings. These maneuvers also can irritate the subacromial space in patients with impingement, and, in the presence of posterior capsular contracture and discomfort, the glenohumeral joint will be localized accordingly. Injection of local anesthetic is an excellent confirmatory test when AC joint pathology is suspected, although the arthritic AC joint can be somewhat difficult to enter successfully. It is helpful to remember that the obliquity of the joint is such that entry is most frequently successful with the needle directed at an angle of variable magnitude from superolateral to inferomedial.[51]

FIGURE 8

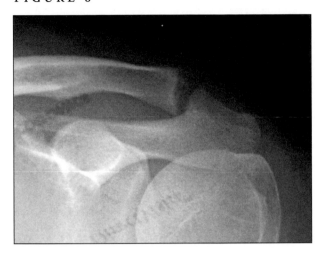

Radiograph showing washed-out appearance of the distal clavicle in distal clavicular osteolysis.

TABLE 6

Shubin-Stein Classification

Grade	MRI Findings
I	Normal
II (Mild)	Capsular distension
III (Moderate)	Joint space narrowing, subacromial fat effacement, marginal osteophytes
IV (Severe)	Marked joint space narrowing, large osteophytes

FIGURE 9

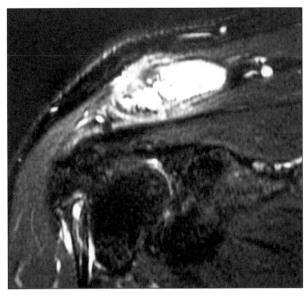

Coronal T2-weighted MRI scan of the AC joint with significant bony edema on both sides of the joint, predictive of symptomatic AC joint arthritis.

Radiographic Evaluation

AP radiographs of the shoulder show typical changes associated with AC joint OA, including joint space narrowing and proliferation of osteophytes. In the presence of distal clavicle osteolysis, the distal end of the clavicle will have a classic washed-out, frequently expansile appearance (Figure 8). In addition to the standard shoulder series, the inferior border and general orientation of the AC joint are nicely profiled on a Zanca projection, which is obtained using a 10° to 15° cranial tilt.[52] Also, the axillary view should be inspected for any AP incongruity if a history of trauma is given, and the outlet view assesses the distal clavicle for inferior spurs.

Arthritic changes commonly are seen in asymptomatic patients, and the presence of degeneration alone is not an indication for treatment.[53] The frequency of radiographic AC joint abnormality can lead to overdiagnosis of AC joint arthritis, especially in the presence of concomitant subacromial pathology. Sequential subacromial and AC joint injection with examination before and after injection is an excellent method for confirming the presence or absence of both entities.

MRI often has been obtained in these patients to evaluate the rotator cuff, and recent literature has shown MRI to be useful in the differentiation of AC pathology, although false-positive findings are common. Stein and associates[54] graded MRI changes of the AC joint and found that severity of changes increased with age, even in asymptomatic patients (Table 6). Further investigation revealed that, when coupled with positive physical findings, bony edema of the AC joint on the T2-weighted images was highly reliable for true AC joint arthritis[55] (Figure 9).

Treatment

Nonsurgical treatment of AC joint arthritis consists of physical therapy to maintain ROM and treat any concomitant impingement. NSAIDs and corticosteroid

FIGURE 10

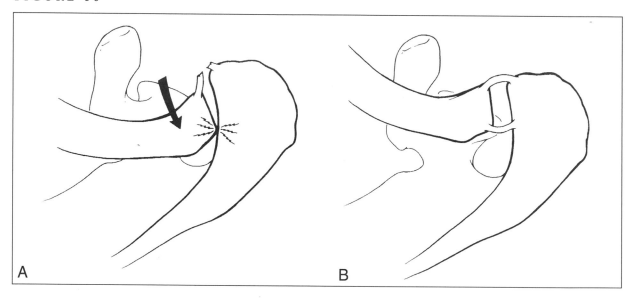

A, Disruption of the superior capsule allows posterior translation and abutment against the acromial base. **B,** Preservation of the superior ligaments maintains AC stability, preventing abutment. *(Reproduced from Flatow EL: The biomechanics of the acromioclavicular, sternoclavicular, and scapulothoracic joints.* Instr Course Lect *1993;42:237-245.)*

injection also are useful, with the latter having diagnostic value.

The eponymous Mumford procedure, reported in 1941, describes open resection of the distal clavicle;[56] Gurd[57] also reported this procedure for treatment of chronic arthritis after AC separation in the same year. Although results of the open Mumford procedure have been uniformly satisfactory, the prominent scar and a subtle loss of strength are identified drawbacks of this open approach.[58-61] Arthroscopic distal clavicle resection was introduced by Johnson[62] in 1981. Arthroscopic resection has been reported to have results equivalent to those of open resection, perhaps with a slightly more rapid recovery in the early postoperative phase,[63,64] as well as resection without violation of the superior AC capsule. This resection has been described with both a superior (direct) approach and a bursal surface (indirect) technique.[48,50,65] Recent information suggests that although both direct and indirect methods are effective, the indirect approach may have a slightly higher success rate and a lower rate of postoperative instability than the direct approach.[66]

Successful outcome is based on performing an even, complete resection of bone with preservation of the superior ligaments; when this is achieved, usually only 5 to 7 mm of distal clavicular resection is necessary.[48] Renfree and associates,[67] reporting a cadaveric study, noted that resection greater than 5 mm in women and 7 mm in men may result in violation of the superior AC capsule. Incompetence of the superior capsule may lead to excessive AP motion, resulting in painful abutment of the clavicle on the acromion despite significant resection of the distal clavicle (Figure 10). Open distal clavicle resection with stabilization is preferred, given a history of grade II or higher AC separation.[6,50] Debski and associates,[68] performing a biomechanical study, reported 30% increased excursion of the AC joint in the AP plane after bursal-sided AC joint resection. Although this finding did not appear to be of clinical significance, the authors theorized that any preexisting injury to other ligaments of the joint may predispose patients to pathologic instability after resection alone.

Technique

We prefer regional anesthesia and beach chair positioning as described previously when performing arthroscopic distal clavicle resection. We use indirect resection

FIGURE 11

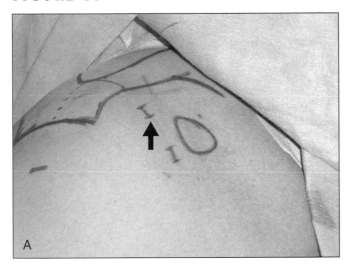
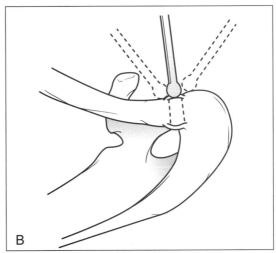

A, Intraoperative view of the right shoulder with high superior portal for distal clavicle resection (*arrow*) just lateral to the coracoid tip. **B,** Placement of the anterior instrument portal either too laterally or medially makes the angle of resection unfavorable, leading either to inadequate resection or asymmetrically excessive resection. The correct portal places the burr directly in line with the distal clavicle.

when intra-articular or subacromial pathology coexists, whereas either the direct or indirect method for isolated AC joint arthritis may be used.

Bursal (Indirect) Approach

Standard arthroscopic distal clavicle resection begins with glenohumeral arthroscopy using a standard posterior portal for the camera. A high anterior working portal is established; precise placement of this portal is crucial if it also is to be used for the distal clavicle resection. This portal is made just under a centimeter lateral and slightly superior to the coracoid process, which ensures two things. First, proper placement avoids injury to the major neurovascular structures, which are medial to the coracoid. Second, placing the anterior portal in line with the AC joint facilitates smooth, even resection of the entire clavicle. Placement of this portal too medial or lateral will cause the resection tool to enter from a poor angle, making adequate resection nearly impossible without cutting a significant amount of bone off either the anteromedial acromion or anterolateral clavicle (Figure 11).

After glenohumeral arthroscopy, the camera cannula is withdrawn and introduced into the subacromial space via the same posterior skin incision. At this point, a lateral portal is placed to facilitate bursectomy and

anterior subacromial decompression as indicated. Subacromial bursectomy generally begins laterally because the bursa tends to be more vascular medially. Once the decompression is completed, the AC joint is identified. A common error when gaining experience with this procedure is to look for the AC joint too posteriorly, which not only is time consuming but also often results in bleeding as the richly vascularized medial bursa is débrided in search of the joint. If anterior portal placement was accurate, a reliable method for finding the AC joint is to drive the arthroscope through the anterior portal and rotate it to view medially, which consistently brings the AC joint into view. Identification is confirmed by applying pressure over the distal clavicle and observing its motion through the arthroscope.

Electrocautery is used to débride the capsule and remaining bursa obscuring the joint. A burr is then introduced through the anterior portal and the resection begins on the anteroinferior corner and is continued circumferentially around the clavicle for a total resection of 8 to 10 mm. The resection may be performed with the camera in either the lateral or the posterior portal. Having an assistant place downward pressure on the distal clavicle will help deliver it into view. Use of a 30° arthroscope may necessitate judicious resection of a portion of the medial acromion to

FIGURE 12

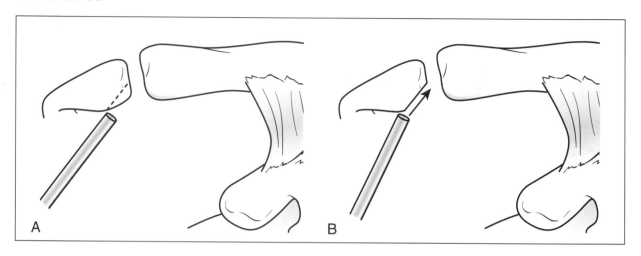

A, Shaded area shows medial acromial undersurface in which resection facilitates visualization of entire distal clavicular surface. **B,** Minimal resection of the medial acromion has allowed even, circumferential resection of the distal clavicle.

FIGURE 13

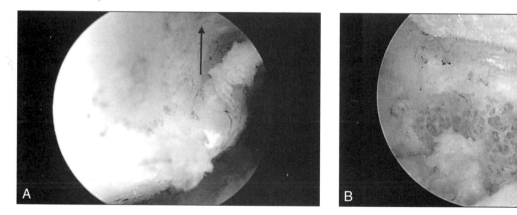

A, Arthroscopic view of the left shoulder from the anterior viewing portal showing resected AC joint with distal clavicle to the left and, above, unresected portion of posterosuperior distal clavicle (*arrow*) that was not visible from the lateral portal. **B,** Arthroscopic view of the left shoulder from the lateral portal shows thorough, even resection of the distal clavicle.

see around the corner of the acromion and visualize the superior aspect of the distal clavicle, which otherwise may be left behind (Figure 12). Care must be taken to avoid disrupting the superior capsule in order to maintain anteroposterior stability of the AC joint.

We prefer to confirm circumferential resection by placing the camera in the anterior portal. If the resection is incomplete, the C-like appearance of the resected distal clavicle with its persistent roof is readily appar-

ent, and the superior aspect must be leveled with the remainder of the distal clavicle resection (Figure 13). In rare instances this step has required insertion of an elevator through the anterior portal to separate the superior AC ligaments from the remnant of clavicle rather than risk injury to these structures with the burr. Alternatively, a portal can be created just off the posterosuperior aspect of the AC joint to complete the resection superiorly.

FIGURE 14

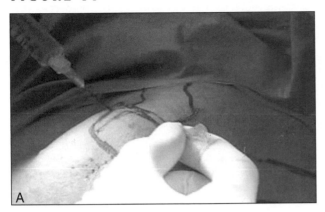
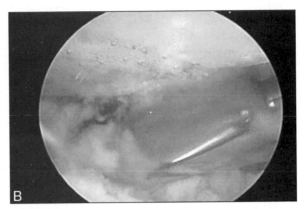

A, Posterolateral intraoperative view of the left shoulder with needle localization of the AC joint for direct arthroscopic resection. **B,** Arthroscopic view of the left AC joint from the anterior viewing portal showing establishment of posterior portal under direct vision during direct arthroscopic resection of the distal clavicle.

Superior (Direct) Approach

The superior (direct) approach is useful in the case of isolated AC joint arthritis in which subacromial and rotator cuff pathology are absent. The major proposed advantage is sparing of the acromion and coracoacromial ligament, which occasionally must be partially resected to gain access to the AC joint from the bursal approach. The joint is localized anteriorly and posteriorly with 18-gauge spinal needles, followed by the establishment of a viewing portal superior to the AC joint just off the anterior margin (generally about 5 mm off the joint margin). This step is followed by placement of an instrument portal posteriorly under direct vision (Figure 14). Placement of portals too close to the AC joint may result in compromise of the superior AC capsule and subsequent instability. A small-joint arthroscope (2.7 mm) often is necessary initially until the joint is opened by preliminary resection. Resection proceeds from anteroinferior to posterosuperior, taking approximately 4 to 5 mm off the distal clavicle and 3 to 4 mm off the medial acromion. The arthroscope and shaver portals usually must be switched by the end of the procedure to complete the resection anteriorly. The small distance between the skin superiorly and the AC joint translates into a favorable angle for resection, facilitating resection of the superior portion of the distal clavicle, which is occasionally difficult using the bursal approach.

Postoperative Management

We prefer to document the distal clavicle resection with an AP radiograph in the recovery room. This surgery is an outpatient procedure. The patient wears a sling for several days to minimize pain, after which passive motion is started and active motion is encouraged. Physical therapy to encourage motion is prescribed as indicated. Strengthening is permitted at 6 weeks.

Results

Success of arthroscopic distal clavicle resection for arthritis and osteolysis has ranged from 83% to 100%.[5-10] Flatow and associates[5] reported 83% satisfactory results after distal clavicle resection via the direct approach for isolated AC pathology. These results were further improved to 93% satisfaction when patients with grade II chronic AC separations were excluded. Levine and associates[48] reported 87.5% good to excellent results following arthroscopic distal clavicle excision from a bursal approach in patients who underwent simultaneous anterior subacromial decompression for impingement. There were three failures; one was a patient with a grade II AC separation, another patient did not receive a complete, even resection of bone, and pain was not relieved in the last patient.

Asymptomatic calcification within the region of resected clavicle is well documented. A recent report of long-term results of arthroscopic distal clavicle excision yielded 100% satisfaction with a mean follow-up of 6 years. Ossification within the area of resected clavicle was reported in 5 of 20 patients, although they were asymptomatic.[7] Similarly favorable long-term results were reported for arthroscopic treatment of distal clavicle osteolysis.[69] Snyder and associates[10] reported 94% good to excellent results in their series of indirect resections; they also noted calcification within the resected space in 16% of patients, several of whom had residual pain postoperatively.

A recent study may indicate slightly superior results of indirect versus direct arthroscopic resection. Levine and associates[66] retrospectively reviewed a series of arthroscopic distal clavicle resections performed from either a direct or indirect approach. In the indirect cohort, 100% success was reached, whereas 90% success was seen in the direct group. Two of the four failures in the direct group required later stabilization procedures for symptomatic anteroposterior laxity, suggesting that the direct approach may place the superior capsule at more risk than the indirect method.

Complications

Complications of arthroscopic distal clavicle resection incident to subacromial arthroscopy generally can occur, including postoperative hematoma and infection, reflex sympathetic dystrophy, and traction neurapraxia. One case of AC fusion after arthroscopic resection has been reported.[70] Anteroposterior instability after the direct approach is a recent finding.[66]

CONCLUSION

Distal clavicle excision is well established as the surgical procedure of choice for AC joint arthritis. Arthroscopic distal clavicle resection has proved to be reproducible and highly effective. Preservation of the superior capsule yields the best results, and a well-performed arthroscopic resection consistently achieves this goal.

Arthroscopy has a limited role in the treatment of glenohumeral arthritis. The gold standard remains total shoulder arthroplasty; nevertheless, arthroscopy is a viable option in the small group of patients who meet the relatively limited indications. Most patients will present at a point beyond which arthroscopy is indicated, but in the carefully selected group with early arthritis, it has proved effective. Although it is apparent that débridement may provide only temporary relief from

the inevitable series of events that occurs in arthritis, it is possible that the combination of surgical débridement with the latest medical therapies may potentiate the effects that each of these therapies would offer alone. By inhibiting the erosive process, pain may be controlled, the need for more aggressive procedures delayed, and bone stock preserved for future index arthroplasty.

REFERENCES

1. Cameron BD, Galatz LM, Ramsey ML, Williams GR, Iannotti JP: Non-prosthetic management of grade IV osteochondral lesions of the glenohumeral joint. *J Shoulder Elbow Surg* 2002;11:25-32.

2. Ogilvie-Harris DJ, Wiley AM: Arthroscopic surgery of the shoulder: A general appraisal. *J Bone Joint Surg Br* 1986;68:201-207.

3. Weinstein DM, Bucchieri JS, Pollock RG, Flatow EL, Bigliani LU: Arthroscopic debridement of the shoulder for osteoarthritis. *Arthroscopy* 2000;16:471-476.

4. Ellman H, Kay SP, Wirth M: Arthroscopic treatment of full-thickness rotator cuff tears: 2- to 7-year follow-up study. *Arthroscopy* 1993;9:195-200.

5. Flatow EL, Duralde XA, Nicholson GP, Pollock RG, Bigliani LU: Arthroscopic resection of the distal clavicle with a superior approach. *J Shoulder Elbow Surg* 1995;4:41-50.

6. Gartsman GM: Arthroscopic resection of the acromioclavicular joint. *Am J Sports Med* 1993;21:71-77.

7. Kay SP, Dragoo JL, Lee R: Long-term results of arthroscopic resection of the distal clavicle with concomitant subacromial decompression. *Arthroscopy* 2003;19:805-809.

8. Jerosch J, Steinbeck J, Schroder M, Castro WH: Arthroscopic resection of the acromioclavicular joint (ARAC). *Knee Surg Sports Traumatol Arthrosc* 1993;1:209-215.

9. Auge WK II, Fischer RA: Arthroscopic distal clavicle resection for isolated atraumatic osteolysis in weight lifters. *Am J Sports Med* 1998;26:189-192.

10. Snyder SJ, Banas MP, Karzel RP: The arthroscopic Mumford procedure: An analysis of results. *Arthroscopy* 1995;11:157-164.

11. Neer CS II: Replacement arthroplasty for glenohumeral osteoarthritis. *J Bone Joint Surg Am* 1974;56:1-13.

12. Booth R: Arthroscopy before arthroplasty: A con or comfort? *J Arthroplasty* 2004;19:2-4.

13. Moseley JB, O'Malley K, Petersen NJ, et al: A controlled trial of arthroscopic surgery for osteoarthritis of the knee. *N Engl J Med* 2002;347:81-88.

14. Scott WN, Clarke HD: Early knee arthritis: The role of arthroscopy. Beneficial or placebo? *Orthopedics* 2003;26:943-944.

15. Ellman H, Harris E, Kay SP: Early degenerative joint disease simulating impingement syndrome: Arthroscopic findings. *Arthroscopy* 1992;8:482-487.

16. Jazrawi L, Sherman O, Hunt S: Arthroscopic management of osteoarthritis of the knee. *J Am Acad Orthop Surg* 2003;11:290.

17. Neer CS II, Watson KC, Stanton FJ: Recent experience in total shoulder replacement. *J Bone Joint Surg Am* 1982;64:319-337.

18. Kellgren JH, Lawrence JS: Radiological assessment of osteoarthritis. *Ann Rheum Dis* 1957;16:494-502.

19. Cofield RH: Arthroscopy of the shoulder. *Mayo Clin Proc* 1983;58:501-508.

20. Lusardi DA, Wirth MA, Wurtz D, et al: Loss of external rotation following anterior capsulorraphy of the shoulder. *J Bone Joint Surg Am* 1993;75:1185-1192.

21. Buckwalter JA, Lane NE, Gordon SL: Excercise as a cause of osteoarthritis, in Kuettner KE, Goldberg VL (eds): *Osteoarthritic Disorders.* Rosemont, IL, American Academy of Orthopaedic Surgeons, 1995, pp 405-417.

22. Buckwalter JA, Martin J: Degenerative joint disease. *Clin Symp* 1995;47:1-32.

23. Mankin HJ: The reaction of articular cartilage to injury and osteoarthritis (first of two parts). *N Engl J Med* 1974;291:1285-1292.

24. Mankin HJ: The reaction of articular cartilage to injury and osteoarthritis (second of two parts). *N Engl J Med* 1974;291:1335-1340.

25. Mankin HJ, Dorfman H, Lippiello L, Zarins A: Biochemical and metabolic abnormalities in articular cartilage from osteo-arthritic human hips: II. Correlation of morphology with biochemical and metabolic data. *J Bone Joint Surg Am* 1971;53:523-537.

26. Outerbridge R: The etiology of chondromalacia patellae. *J Bone Joint Surg Br* 1961;43:752-759.

27. Myers SL, Flusser D, Brandt KD, Heck DA: Prevalence of cartilage shards in synovium and their association with synovitis in patients with early and endstage osteoarthritis. *J Rheumatol* 1992;19:1247-1251.

28. Homandberg GA, Meyers R, Williams JM: Intraarticular injection of fibronectin fragments causes severe depletion of cartilage proteoglycans in vivo. *J Rheumatol* 1993;20:1378-1382.

29. Steadman JR, Briggs KK, Rodrigo JJ, Kocher MS, Gill TJ, Rodkey WG: Outcomes of microfracture for traumatic chondral defects of the knee: Average 11-year follow-up. *Arthroscopy* 2003;19:477-484.

30. Siebold R, Lichtenberg S, Habermeyer P: Combination of microfracture and periostal-flap for the treatment of focal full thickness articular cartilage lesions of the shoulder: A prospective study. *Knee Surg Sports Traumatol Arthrosc* 2003;11:183-189.

31. Johnson LL: Arthroscopic abrasion arthroplasty historical and pathologic perspective: Present status. *Arthroscopy* 1986;2:54-69.

32. Steadman JR, Rodkey WA, Singleton SB, Briggs KK: Microfracture technique for full thickness chondral defects: Technique and clinical results. *Oper Tech Orthop* 1997;7:300-307.

33. Schenck RC, Iannotti JP: Prosthetic arthroplasty for glenohumeral arthritis with an intact or repairable rotator cuff: Indications, techniques, and results, in Iannotti JP, Williams GR (eds): *Disorders of the Shoulder: Diagnosis and Management.* Philadelphia, PA, Lippincott, Williams & Wilkins, 1999, pp 521-558.

34. Friedman RJ, Thornhill TS, Thomas WH, Sledge CB: Non-constrained total shoulder replacement in patients who have rheumatoid arthritis and class-IV function. *J Bone Joint Surg Am* 1989;71:494-498.

35. Cohen S, Jones R: An evaluation of the efficacy of arthroscopic synovectomy of the knee in rheumatoid arthritis: 12-24 month results. *J Rheumatol* 1987;14:452-455.

36. Wilkinson MC: Synovectomy for rheumatoid arthritis. *Clin Orthop Relat Res* 1974;100:125-142.

37. Morrey BF, Adams RA: Semiconstrained arthroplasty for the treatment of rheumatoid arthritis of the elbow. *J Bone Joint Surg Am* 1992;74:479-490.

38. Simpson NS: Extra-glenohumeral joint shoulder surgery in rheumatoid arthritis: The role of bursectomy, acromioplasty, and distal clavicle excision. *J Shoulder Elbow Surg* 1994;3:66-69.

39. Hawkins RJ, Angelo RL: Glenohumeral osteoarthrosis: A late complication of the Putti-Platt repair. *J Bone Joint Surg Am* 1990;72:1193-1197.

40. Petty DH, Jazrawi LM, Estrada LS, Andrews JR: Glenohumeral chondrolysis after shoulder arthroscopy: Case reports and review of the literature. *Am J Sports Med* 2004;32:509-515.

41. Levine WN, Bigliani LU, Ahmad CS: Thermal capsulorrhaphy. *Orthopedics* 2004;27:823-826.

42. Levine WN, Clark AM Jr, D'Alessandro DF, Yamaguchi K: Chondrolysis following arthroscopic thermal capsulorrhaphy for shoulder instability: A case report. *J Bone Joint Surg Am* 2005;87:616-621.

43. O'Driscoll SW: Arthroscopic glenoidplasty and osteocapsular arthroplasty for advanced glenohumeral osteoarthritis. *67th Annual Meeting Proceedings.* Rosemont, IL, American Academy of Orthopaedic Surgeons, 2000, pp 193-195.

44. Morgan CD, Casscells CD: Arthroscopic-assisted glenohumeral arthrodesis. *Arthroscopy* 1992;8:262-266.

45. Fukuda K, Craig EV, An KN, Cofield RH, Chao EY: Biomechanical study of the ligamentous system of the

acromioclavicular joint. *J Bone Joint Surg Am* 1986;68:434-440.

46. Codman E: Rupture of the supraspinatus tendon, in Codman EA: *The Shoulder*. Brooklyn, NY, G Miller & Co, 1934, pp 123-177.

47. Fischer BW, Gross RM, McCarthy JA, Arroyo JS: Incidence of acromioclavicular joint complications after arthroscopic subacromial decompression. *Arthroscopy* 1999;15:241-248.

48. Levine WN, Barron OA, Yamaguchi K, Pollock RG, Flatow EL, Bigliani LU: Arthroscopic distal clavicle resection from a bursal approach. *Arthroscopy* 1998;14: 52-56.

49. Cahill B: Osteolysis of the distal part of the clavicle in male athletes. *J Bone Joint Surg Am* 1982;64:1053-1058.

50. Bigliani LU, Nicholson GP, Flatow EL: Arthroscopic resection of the distal clavicle. *Orthop Clin North Am* 1993;24:133-141.

51. DePalma A: *Surgery of the Shoulder*, ed 2, Philadelphia, PA, JB Lipincott, 1973.

52. Zanca P: Shoulder pain: Involvement of the acromioclavicular joint (analysis of 1000 cases). *Am J Roentgenol Radium Ther Nucl Med* 1971;112:493-506.

53. DePalma A: *Degenerative Changes of the Sternoclavicular and Acromioclavicular Joints in Various Decades*. Springfield, IL, CC Thomas, 1957.

54. Stein BE, Wiater JM, Pfaff HC, Bigliani LU, Levine WN: Detection of acromioclavicular joint pathology in asymptomatic shoulders with magnetic resonance imaging. *J Shoulder Elbow Surg* 2001;10:204-208.

55. Shubin Stein BE, Ahmad CS, Pfaff CH, Bigliani LU, Levine WN: A comparison of MRI findings of the acromioclavicular joint in symptomatic versus asymptomatic patients. *J Shoulder Elbow Surg* 2006;15:56-59.

56. Mumford E: Acromioclavicular dislocation: A new operative treatment. *J Bone Joint Surg Am* 1941;23:799-802.

57. Gurd F: The treatment of complete dislocation of the outer end of the clavicle: An hitherto undescribed operation. *Ann Surg* 1941;113:1094-1098.

58. Taft TN, Wilson FC, Oglesby JW: Dislocation of the acromioclavicular joint. An end-result study. *J Bone Joint Surg Am* 1987;69:1045-1051.

59. Cook FF, Tibone JE: The Mumford procedure in athletes: An objective analysis of function. *Am J Sports Med* 1988;16:97-100.

60. Petersson CJ: Resection of the lateral end of the clavicle: A 3 to 30-year follow-up. *Acta Orthop Scand* 1983;54:904-907.

61. Walsh WM: Peterson DA, Shelton G, Neumann RD, Shoulder strength following acromioclavicular injury. *Am J Sports Med* 1985;13:153-158.

62. Johnson L: *Diagnostic and Surgical Arthroscopy*. St Louis, MO, CV Mosby, 1981.

63. Sachs RA, Stone ML, Devine S: Open vs arthroscopic acromioplasty: A prospective, randomized study. *Arthroscopy* 1994;10:248-254.

64. Flatow EL, Cordasco FA, Bigliani LU: Arthroscopic resection of the outer end of the clavicle from a superior approach: A critical, quantitative, radiographic assessment of bone removal. *Arthroscopy* 1992;8:55-64.

65. Flatow EL, Duralde XA, Nicholson GP, Pollock RG, Bigliani LU: Arthroscopic resection of the distal clavicle with a superior approach. *J Shoulder Elbow Surg* 1995;4:41-50.

66. Levine WN, Soong M, Ahmad CS, Blaine TA, Bigliani LU: Arthroscopic distal clavicle resection: A comparison of direct and bursal approaches. *Arthroscopy* 2006;22:516-520.

67. Renfree KJ, Riley MK, Wheeler D, Hentz JG, Wright TW: Ligamentous anatomy of the distal clavicle. *J Shoulder Elbow Surg* 2003;12:355-359.

68. Debski RE, Fenwick JA, Vangura A Jr, Fu FH, Woo SL, Rodosky MW: Effect of arthroscopic procedures on the acromioclavicular joint. *Clin Orthop Relat Res* 2003;406: 89-96.

69. Zawadsky M, Marra G, Wiater JM, et al: Osteolysis of the distal clavicle: Long-term results of arthroscopic resection. *Arthroscopy* 2000;16:600-605.

70. Tytherleigh-Strong G, Gill J, Sforza G, Copeland S, Levy O: Reossification and fusion across the acromioclavicular joint after arthroscopic acromioplasty and distal clavicle resection. *Arthroscopy* 2001;17:E36.

CHAPTER 7

COMPLICATIONS OF ARTHROSCOPIC SHOULDER SURGERY

MARSHALL A. KUREMSKY, MD
PATRICK M. CONNOR, MD
DONALD F. D'ALESSANDRO, MD

The number of arthroscopic shoulder surgeries has risen dramatically over the past 15 years, and consequently, the number and type of associated complications have increased significantly. Recognizing the potential complications and knowing how to treat them is of critical importance. Despite the large number of arthroscopic shoulder surgeries performed by both upper extremity specialists and general orthopaedists, published information on the numerous potential complications of shoulder arthroscopy is limited.[1-8]

The first review articles included a study of 14,329 arthroscopies performed by members of the Arthroscopy Association of North America; this review reported that the highest rate of complications occurred in procedures using staple capsulorrhaphy (5.3%) and the lowest rate occurred in subacromial surgery (0.76%).[1] A later study by Small[2] analyzed the results of 21 experienced arthroscopists from various centers and reported a complication rate of 0.7% after shoulder arthroscopy, with the highest incidences associated with staple capsulorrhaphy (3.3%) and anterior acromioplasty (1.1%). Reports of several other series focusing on complications after shoulder arthroscopy have been subsequently published.[3-10] In this chapter we focus on the type of complications associated with arthroscopic shoulder surgery and discuss means by which their incidence can be minimized. As Berjano and associates[3] and Bigliani and associates[4] have noted, underreporting of complications makes true incidence determinations difficult and can disrupt or delay the dissemination of useful continuing education. Furthermore, the definition of complications can vary widely. For example, Berjano and associates[3] exclude postoperative stiffness as a complication of shoulder arthroscopy, whereas other authors include it in their reports.[4]

The purpose of this chapter is to raise awareness of complications related to arthroscopic shoulder surgery. Although some of these complications may be unavoidable, a high index of suspicion may prove critical in their evaluation and management should they arise. Most complications, however, can be prevented by appropriate caution, experience, technical expertise, and patient selection.

ANESTHESIA, MEDICAL, AND GENERAL SURGICAL COMPLICATIONS

Anesthesia Concerns

Complications associated with general and regional (interscalene block) anesthesia are rare but potentially quite serious. Potential complications of general anesthesia have been recognized for a long time, but a newer subset of case-specific complications now exists. Several anecdotal reports, covering tracheal compression,[11] pneumothorax,[12] epinephrine-induced arrhythmia,[13] and negative-pressure pulmonary edema,[14] have been published. Interscalene blocks can be associated with phrenic nerve paralysis and neurologic injury that is either temporary or permanent.[6] Most of these reports are of small series of specific complications that, in general, appear to be uncommon.

Patient Positioning

It has been postulated that the lateral decubitus position may lead to significant fluid accumulation in the soft tissues of the neck via gravity.[11] In addition, a 10% to 30% incidence of injury to the brachial plexus has been reported by some authors.[4,15,16] These injuries usually are transient neurapraxias secondary to overstretching that resolve over time. Pitman and associates[15] found legitimate potential for neurologic damage while performing shoulder arthroscopy on patients in the lateral decubitus position. These lesions most commonly took the form of subclinical neurapraxias resulting from a combination of traction, arm positioning, and joint distention. The musculocutaneous nerve proved to be at most risk for injury because it may be stretched in positions of traction and abduction.

The beach chair position results in more lower extremity venous pooling than the lateral decubitus position, causing theoretical concern for deep venous thrombosis (DVT), as well as for hypotension and cerebrovascular accident in predisposed patients with severe hypertension or other medical comorbidities. Advantages of this position include reductions in the possibility of traction neurapraxias, potential for continuous repositioning of the arm in all planes if necessary for optimum visualization, and ease of conversion to an open procedure if indicated.

A patient who is improperly positioned in the lateral decubitus position may experience femoral cutaneous nerve palsies; similarly, bony prominences along the wrist and forearm should be protected. Usually these neurapraxias resolve spontaneously, but they can be avoided with attention to detail by both the surgeon and the anesthesia team when positioning the patient. Although patient positioning ultimately is determined according to surgeon preference, knowledge of potential position-specific complications can be helpful.

Infection

Postoperative infection rates for shoulder arthroscopy are fortunately quite low, with reports citing rates from 0.04% to 3.4%.[4,17,18] In practice, most studies report rates well below 1%. Armstrong and Bolding[19] reviewed a consecutive series of arthroscopies after several instances of postarthroscopic septic arthritis were identified at a small surgical center. They concluded that the increased rate seen at that particular institution was caused partly by contamination of electrocardiogram cables with *Pseudomonas aeruginosa* and partly by inadequate procedures to disinfect the arthroscopic equipment. The use of perioperative antibiotic prophylaxis with a first-generation cephalosporin is considered important for decreasing the risk of postoperative infection. Appropriate synovial concentrations are attained following a standard dose of 1 g administered 30 to 60 minutes preoperatively; with this, a fourfold reduction in the infection rate can be expected.[4,18] Johnson and associates[17] reported that disinfecting arthroscopic surgical instruments with 2% glutaraldehyde has proved to be quick, affordable, and effective, with an infection rate of 0.04% in more than 12,500 arthroscopic procedures.

Air Extravasation

Lee and associates[20] reported on three patients who sustained extensive subcutaneous emphysema and pneumomediastinum after undergoing shoulder arthroscopy and subacromial decompression (SAD) for impingement. A large pneumothorax developed in two of these patients, and both required insertion of chest tubes. All three patients eventually recovered uneventfully. These authors' proposed mechanism involved air extravasation from one of the portals when the infusion pump and power shaver with suction were turned on simultaneously. Lau[21] also reported subcutaneous emphysema and pneumomediastinum resulting from shoulder arthroscopy. Dietzel and Ciullo[12] reported spontaneous pneumothorax in four patients after shoulder arthroscopy. All four had a history of smoking, and two of the four had a history of asthma. These authors ultimately recommended that all patients with a substantive smoking history or known pulmonary disease undergo preoperative chest radiographs and that consideration be given to the use of interscalene block anesthesia rather than general endotracheal anesthesia to avoid positive-pressure ventilation.

Air Embolism

Although rare, venous air embolism may occur during any surgical procedure in which the surgical site is above the level of the heart and noncollapsible veins are exposed to atmospheric pressure, or if air or another gas is placed under pressure into a body cavity. Hegde and Avatgere[22] postulate that possible mechanisms associated with development of a venous air embolism during arthroscopy include injection of air into the joint itself, in which the air can enter venous sinuses as a result of very high intra-articular pressures, or accidental injection of air into a vein in the joint. Clinically significant venous air embolism manifests as bronchospasm, hypoxemia, hypercapnia, decreased end-tidal carbon dioxide, and hypotension.[22] Transesophageal echocardiogram is the most sensitive monitor for early detection. Fatal pulmonary air embolism has been reported during knee arthroscopy,[23,24] and venous air embolism during shoulder arthroscopy also has been reported.[25] In the event of suspected or known air embolism, it is imperative to rapidly proceed through a treatment algorithm (Trendelenburg positioning, rotating the patient onto the side, close communication with the anesthesia department, intravenous fluids, consideration to aborting the case, and so forth) to protect the patient.

Thromboembolism

A rare, but serious, consequence of arthroscopic shoulder surgery is DVT and subsequent pulmonary embolus. Reported cases are few. Burkhart reported a single case of complete thrombosis of the basilic and innominate vein after labral débridement; this patient was later found to have Hodgkin's disease.[26] Polzhofer and associates[27] reported a case of isolated DVT after shoulder arthroscopy. In the absence of discrete information that can be used to attribute the etiology of this complication, these authors note that irritation of the subclavian vein caused by compression from the motor-driven shaver represents a likely cause.

Cardiovascular Sequelae

As noted, patient positioning in the beach chair position may decrease venous return and, therefore, ventricular volume; similarly overzealous use of intravenous fluids may lead to bladder distention and discomfort.[28] Use of epinephrine in irrigation fluid or as a local anesthetic can increase ventricular contractility.

GENERAL COMPLICATIONS RELATED TO SHOULDER ARTHROSCOPY

Portal Placement

Several routine portals have been described for shoulder arthroscopy. The standard posterior portal,[29] central anterior portal,[30] and lateral subacromial portal are relatively safe but are not without risk of injury to underlying neurovascular structures. If the posterior portal is placed too medially and superiorly, the suprascapular nerve may be injured. If it is placed too inferiorly, the axillary nerve and posterior humeral circumflex artery may be injured.[31] Cadaveric dissections by Matthews and associates[30] and Flatow and associates[32] have shown that an anterosuperior portal made lateral to the coracoid process protects the patient from iatrogenic damage to structures located more medially. Davidson and Tibone[33] described an anteroinferior portal in the 5 o'clock position that leaves the musculocutaneous nerve an average of 22 mm and the axillary nerve an average of 24 mm away from the portal.

Irrigation Fluid, Visualization, and Bleeding

Visual clarity of arthroscopic procedures often is compromised by intra-articular or subacromial bleeding, necessitating high pressure and flow of irrigation fluid. Electrocautery has helped decrease the incidence of bleeding complications according to Bigliani and associates.[4] Contrary to knee arthroscopy, procedures in the subacromial space do not have the benefit of a pneumatic tourniquet or a fluid-restricting structure such as a synovial lining. Suggested means to improve arthroscopic visualization include the use of hypotensive anesthesia, the use of coagulation, maintaining irrigation fluids at the proper height, and the use of cold irrigation fluid.[4,34-36] In a prospective randomized study by Jensen and associates,[37] addition of epinephrine to irrigation fluid reduced intra-articular bleeding, improved visual clarity, and was not associated with any adverse cardiovascular effects related to heart rate or blood pressure. Other relevant findings were reported by Morrison and associates[38] in a study exploring the relationship of subacromial space pressure, blood pressure, and visual clarity during SAD. Clarity can be improved by increasing flow rates or by manipulating the pressure of the irrigation fluid, but this is done at the potential expense of fluid extravasation into the surrounding tissues. They reported that an average pressure difference of 49 mm Hg between the patient's systolic blood pressure and the subacromial space pressure was enough to achieve adequate visualization. The historic use of 1.5% glycine in irrigation solutions has all but been abandoned because of reports in the urologic and orthopaedic literature of transient postoperative blindness.[39]

Fluid Extravasation

Fluid extravasation into the shoulder girdle and chest is a recognized feature of shoulder arthroscopy. Deltoid muscle pressures increase during arthroscopy, particularly in procedures involving the subacromial space because it is not enclosed within a capsule. Although intramuscular pressures decrease shortly after surgery, clinical swelling may persist for some time with local symptoms.[40,41] Problems associated with excess swelling include increased difficulty with the procedure, a change in the preoperative location of bony landmarks, or added difficulty if converting to an open or mini-open procedure. To protect against unforeseen intraoperative complications associated with swelling, Bigliani and associates[4] recommend that all landmarks and portals be well marked before beginning the procedure for better orientation in the event of massive edema. Additional steps to avoid excess swelling include maintaining an efficient pace of surgery, particularly within the subacromial space, and a stepwise transition to all-arthroscopic procedures, particularly for the less experienced arthroscopic surgeon.[42]

Although local swelling is the most common problem of prolonged shoulder arthroscopy, more severe consequences have been reported. Hynson and associates[43] reported on the care of a patient who suddenly developed complete airway obstruction and severe respiratory distress while undergoing routine shoulder arthroscopy in the lateral decubitus position with interscalene block anesthesia. After the procedure was stopped, the patient was emergently intubated and stabilized. Their differential diagnosis also included airway compression from a hematoma, tension pneumothorax, phrenic nerve paralysis, or anaphylaxis. These same authors additionally

reported an increase in neck circumference of up to 5 cm after routine shoulder arthroscopy.[43]

Vascular Injury

Vascular injuries are rare and usually involve laceration of the cephalic vein from the anterior portal, causing hematoma. Cameron[44] reported on the development of a venous pseudoaneurysm caused by unintentional laceration of a high-pressure cephalic vein without subsequent proper ligation in a renal dialysis patient. The author recommends selecting alternatives to anterior portal placement in the uncommon instance of upper extremity arteriovenous fistula, if possible.

Nerve Injury

Nerve injury is one of the most common complications associated with shoulder arthroscopy; rates from 0 to 30% have been reported.[15,16,29,45,46] Nerves may be injured in any number of ways: strain injury from traction, improper positioning leading to neurapraxias, or direct injury during portal placement or during the surgical procedure itself.[5,47,48] Reports of injuries to specific peripheral nerves have included the axillary,[1] musculocutaneous,[15,29,34] median,[49] and radial nerves.[15] These specific peripheral nerves are at particular risk depending on the surgical procedure being performed and will be discussed individually in subsequent sections.

A 20% incidence of transient paresthesias in the upper extremity was reported after shoulder arthroscopy when traction was used.[50] Although most of these neurapraxias heal with time, one patient was reported to have median nerve palsy that did not recover, necessitating tendon transfers.[30] In a review of neurologic complications of shoulder arthroscopy, Rodeo and associates[48] reported that most were neurapraxias and may have been caused by a variety of mechanisms including direct injury, fluid extravasation causing compression, a tourniquet effect from wrapping the upper extremity, and reflex sympathetic dystrophy. Segmuller and associates[45] reported that 7% of 304 patients undergoing arthroscopy in the lateral decubitus position had a sensory deficit at 2 weeks postoperatively, and 3% had a persistent deficit at a follow-up of 8 months. Klein and associates[16] measured cadaveric plexus strain in the lateral decubitus position and found that two positions during arthroscopy—45° of forward flexion and either 0° or 90° of abduction—maximized visibility and minimized strain on the plexus. Pitman and associates[15] monitored somatosensory evoked potentials in the lateral decubitus position and reported that longitudinal traction less than 12 lb or vertical traction less than 7 lb was not associated with a decrease in brachial plexus somatosensory-evoked potentials.

Although most reported neurologic complications following shoulder arthroscopy have occurred in patients in the lateral decubitus position, a hypoglossal nerve palsy reported in a patient in the beach chair position was believed to be caused by patient positioning.[51] Mohammed and associates[52] reported on three patients with nerve injuries after arthroscopy in the lateral decubitus position. Two patients sustained injury to the medial pectoral nerve, and one patient had injury to the anterior interosseous nerve. The precise mechanism of injury was unknown, but the authors speculate that possible causes include forearm compression from the arm compression sleeve, neurologic injury from the interscalene block, brachial neuritis, or other unknown factors. Ellman[49] reported transient neurologic injury in three patients secondary to suboptimal padding with wrist traction. Reflex sympathetic dystrophy is a rare lesion that is seen infrequently after shoulder arthroscopy.[2,6]

Iatrogenic Tendon Injury

Norwood and Fowler[53] reported four instances of iatrogenic rotator cuff injury after shoulder arthroscopy in young athletes; all of these injuries were visualized first with arthrography then confirmed by direct visualization at the time of repair. The authors warned against trocar insertion through the avascular portion of the tendon during placement of the posterior portal and suggested avoiding substantial external rotation of the extremity during trocar placement. If uncomplicated shoulder arthroscopy fails to relieve symptoms, it is important to consider iatrogenic rotator cuff tear in the differential diagnosis. Souryal and Baker[54] studied the supraclavicular fossa portal in a series of cadavers and found no penetration of the rotator cuff when the arm was in 0° to 30° of abduction. Increased penetration of the rotator cuff tendon was seen with increasing abduction, however. At 90° of abduction, the trocar penetrated all rotator cuffs in

their cadaver models. Bonsell[55] reported a patient with a deltoid detachment that was recognized during shoulder arthroscopy and subsequently repaired during open surgery.

Surgeons have questioned whether the midlateral acromial portal (portal of Wilmington), often used for SLAP (superior labrum anterior and posterior) lesion repairs, results in injury to the supraspinatus. In our experience, this portal usually traverses the musculotendinous junction of the supraspinatus and does not compromise this important rotator cuff muscle's function or cause lasting discomfort.

Articular Cartilage Injury

Articular cartilage scuffing may occur during instrument insertion and use or when using various arthroscopic instruments such as suture passing devices and drills. McFarland and associates[5] note that both chondral damage and humeral head penetration are possible when the trocar forcefully enters the glenohumeral joint. Obviously, avoiding articular cartilage injury is imperative, and these injuries can be minimized with careful, meticulous technique and patience. Using a blunt trocar also may be helpful to minimize the consequences of inadvertent excess penetration.

Skin Injury

Mohammed and associates[52] reported three patients with iatrogenic thermal injury from use of electrocautery. They postulated that two patients sustained injury from overheated irrigation fluid when the fluid volume and flow were low during changing of the fluid bags with the electrocautery still in use. Both wounds were superficial and healed uneventfully. In the other patient, the insulated diathermy sleeve was in contact with the skin for more than 2 minutes, resulting in a full-thickness burn that was excised uneventfully. The authors also reported two instances of skin ischemia after shoulder arthroscopy, most likely stemming from marked swelling and fluid extravasation. In one patient the ischemia progressed to necrosis, requiring split-thickness skin grafts. The authors concluded that impaired skin perfusion may occur secondary to mechanical compression of skin vessels from increased tissue pressure and vasoconstriction caused by epinephrine in irrigation fluid.

Stiffness

Stiffness is a common and troublesome postoperative complication that leads to morbidity and dissatisfaction for both patient and surgeon. Incidence rates as high as 15% have been cited,[8] but the incidence of clinically significant stiffness is most likely far less. The type of repair or procedure being performed to address the underlying pathology often foreshadows and characterizes the stiffness that may follow. For example, the postoperative "captured shoulder" frequently results from extensive subacromial scar after subacromial surgery,[56] and internal rotation contractures frequently may develop in patients undergoing surgery for anterior instability, particularly if prolonged immobilization in a sling and swathe is used.[6] Physical therapy represents the first line of prevention as well as early treatment of this complication. Manipulation with arthroscopic release is an effective and accepted therapeutic option for recalcitrant shoulders and is not associated with the development of recurrent instability, even in the patient with a primary diagnosis of instability.[56,57] External rotation is often the most difficult to restore. Release and débridement of the scar lateral to the coracoid, especially the coracohumeral ligament, is essential to achieve a successful outcome.

Learning Curve

Bigliani and associates[4] note that many of the general complications associated with shoulder arthroscopy may be attributable to the learning curve needed to familiarize the surgeon with all the technical aspects involved in shoulder arthroscopy. Most orthopaedic surgery residency training programs augment the clinical sports medicine and shoulder surgery experiences of their trainees with arthroscopic surgical skills laboratories. Rockwood[58] and Yamaguchi and associates[42] urge those surgeons who may have less experience in arthroscopy at the start of their practice to perform initial diagnostic shoulder arthroscopy followed by open procedures before attempting more difficult arthroscopic repairs, a tactic previously used by knee arthroscopists.

Miscellaneous

Muller and Landsiedl[59] reported on over 800 shoulder arthroscopic procedures with a complication rate of 5.8%. Complications included stiffness, neurologic injury, instrument breakage, drug allergy, and infection.

The authors found an association between complication rates and duration of the surgery. Moran and Warren[60] reported formation of a synovial cyst from the posterior portal that later required excision after arthroscopic shoulder surgery.

COMPLICATIONS OF SPECIFIC ARTHROSCOPIC PROCEDURES

As shoulder arthroscopy has advanced, specific arthroscopic procedures have been developed with the goal of achieving clinical outcomes comparable to those of the corresponding open procedures. In this section failures are distinguished from complications because the former is addressed in detail in other chapters of this monograph. This section focuses more on specific technical complications that are unique to particular procedures in shoulder arthroscopy.

Instability Surgery and Labral Repairs

Metallic staple fixation for instability repair has fallen out of favor as a result of high complication rates related to the hardware. Complications include impingement from an articular staple reported by Matthews and associates,[61] and an 11% recurrence rate resulting from staple loosening, bending, or breaking reported by Hawkins.[35] Suture anchors and screws have become preferred fixation devices for repair.

The potential for nerve injury in arthroscopic stabilization is greater than in open repair because of the proximity to nerves around the joint of anterior and posterior portals used for accessing the capsule and labrum.[61-63] The suprascapular nerve, descending along the posterior glenoid neck, is at risk for injury during glenohumeral arthroscopy, and permanent injury has been reported.[64,65] Bigliani and associates[66] conducted an anatomic study to determine a safe zone for drilling and suturing during anterior capsular suture repair. The axillary nerve may be injured as it courses through the quadrangular space if the instruments are placed too inferiorly; Bryan and associates[67] have shown that the main trunk of the axillary nerve is 0.5 to 2.5 cm inferior to the position of the standard posterior portal. The musculocutaneous nerve also may be injured while entering the coracobrachial muscles below the coracoid process if the anterior portal is placed too inferiorly or medially with respect to the coracoid process.[32]

FIGURE 1

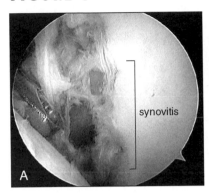 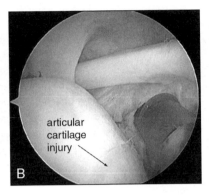 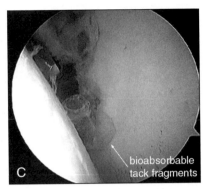

Synovitis **(A)** and articular cartilage injury **(B)** resulting from fragments of retained, undissolved bioabsorbable tacks **(C)** used for labral repair.

Numerous case reports have documented complications related to the placement of labral tacks or suture anchors, both metallic and bioabsorbable. The transglenoid repair technique also has been associated with fistula and cyst formation and intrathoracic penetration with a Beath pin.[60,68] Tack capsulorrhaphy has been associated with morbid synovitis related to tack degradation products.[69] Shaffer and Tibone[6] reviewed literature associated with complications of arthroscopic instability repair, reporting only that recurrence rates from the studies they reviewed showed wide variation in results even when similar surgical techniques were used. Rhee and associates[70] reported on five patients with glenohumeral arthropathy secondary to misplaced suture anchors at the time of arthroscopic anterior glenohumeral stabilization. In their series, all patients reported sharp pain and catching during early rehabilitation as soon as range-of-motion exercises were initiated; this symptom is indicative of iatrogenic misplacement of anchors. Loose anchors, which may migrate but remain partially inserted into bone, are more often associated with a clinically symptom-free interval between surgery and presentation of symptoms. These authors caution that delay in the recognition of migration, loosening, misplacement, or device breakage may lead to anchor-induced glenohumeral arthropathy. Matthews and associates[61] reported that humeral head impingement caused articular cartilage damage in 1 of 25 shoulders that underwent arthroscopic staple capsulorrhaphy for anterior instability. Freehill and associates[71] reported on 10 patients who had clinically significant synovitis after arthroscopic stabilization with poly-L-lactic acid implants. Nine patients had gross implant debris at repeat arthroscopy, and three developed full-thickness chondral defects involving the humeral head and glenoid. They attributed the delayed onset of pain and stiffness to extensive foreign body reactions to crystalline material. Retained bioabsorbable tack fragments may result in synovitis and articular cartilage injury (Figure 1). Petty and associates[72] described three instances of spontaneous idiopathic glenohumeral chondrolysis after routine shoulder arthroscopy in young throwing athletes; the patients underwent repeat arthroscopy for débridement and were allowed to return to their activities as tolerated.

Thermal Capsulorrhaphy

Reports on thermal capsulorrhaphy have documented a variety of complications, including axillary nerve injury, capsular ablation, adhesive capsulitis, recurrent instability, and catastrophic chondrolysis of the entire glenohumeral joint.[6] D'Alessandro and associates[73] reviewed prospectively gathered data on thermal capsulorrhaphy for instability at a follow-up of 2 to 5 years. They found successful clinical results in only 63% of all patients, with the best results in patients with traumatic shoulder dislocations (75% excellent or satisfactory) and the poorest results in patients with multidirectional instability (55% excellent or satisfactory). Complications included axillary nerve sensory dysesthesias (14% of patients), all of which resolved spontaneously and completely by 3 months, and adhesive capsulitis in one

FIGURE 2

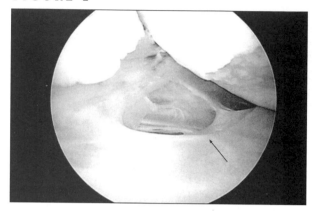

Thin, perforated capsule *(arrow)* found at the time of repeat arthroscopy in a patient with multidirectional instability who previously was treated with thermal capsulorrhaphy.

patient who later required arthroscopic release. The authors also believe there was an experience-related decrease in complications.

Wong and Williams[74] also reviewed complications of thermal capsulorrhaphy. They found a 1.4% rate of axillary nerve injury, which resolved spontaneously in most patients, and a higher associated rate of capsular insufficiency when recurrent instability occurred. They also observed differences in the prevalence of axillary nerve injury when different devices were used: 0.3% after laser, 1.48% after monopolar, and 1.43% after bipolar radiofrequency.

Several authors have identified capsular attenuation and even complete defects after thermal capsulorrhaphy.[74,75] Performing revision open procedures after thermal capsulorrhaphy because of thin, attenuated capsular tissue can be difficult. In one patient, ablation of a portion of capsule resulted in a complete capsular defect (Figure 2). The ability to salvage a failed thermal shrinkage with an open stabilization procedure is an important consideration. Unfortunately, D'Alessandro and associates[73] achieved satisfactory clinical results with revision open capsular shift for failed thermal capsulorrhaphy in only 50% of patients (5 of 10).

Hanypsiak and associates[76] reported on two young male athletes who sustained complete tears of the long head of the biceps tendon with subsequent "Popeye" deformity within 3 months of thermal capsulorrhaphy.

We have encountered several instances of complete loss of the entire humeral and glenoid articular cartilage surfaces, a condition called chondrolysis, after thermal capsulorrhaphy. Presumably, during the course of the procedure, sustained temperature elevation of the arthroscopic fluid in the glenohumeral joint resulted in significant chondrocyte death that initiated a cascade of cartilage degradation and destruction (Figure 3). Unfortunately, this devastating complication usually occurs in young patients who subsequently develop severe stiffness and pain. Attempts at manipulation and arthroscopic release in this setting have not resulted in improved function or lasting pain relief. Humeral resurfacing or hemiarthroplasty combined with placement of an interpositional lateral meniscal allograft has been beneficial for these patients, but long-term outcomes are unknown (Figure 4).

In light of the relatively high failure rates of thermal capsulorrhaphy for shoulder instability and the problematic potential nerve and articular cartilage complications, we have abandoned using this procedure in our practice.

Subacromial Decompression and Distal Clavicle Resection

With overall complication rates of 0.76%[1] and 0.25%,[2] subacromial surgery has the fewest reported complications of any particular arthroscopic procedures. The single most commonly reported cause of failed arthroscopic acromioplasty is inadequate acromial resection.[6,77] To combat this issue, Matthews and Blue[77] developed a detailed plan for preoperative and intraoperative care. Irrigation fluid with epinephrine, electrocautery, and proper hydrostatic pressure can all contribute to thorough hemostasis to allow for enhanced visualization during acromioplasty.[6,77]

In addition to suboptimal SAD, other reported complications include spur regrowth, distal clavicle osteolysis, and heterotopic ossification.[52,78-80] Berg and associates[78] reported on complications of arthroscopic SAD, including traction neuropathy or hematoma,[49] and infection, reflex sympathetic dystrophy, or acromial fracture.[81] In their series, 10 patients underwent arthroscopic SAD and heterotopic bone developed postoperatively, which caused symptoms of recurrent impingement in eight; these authors recommend prophylaxis with indomethacin or radiation therapy in patients at risk for heterotopic bone, such as individu-

FIGURE 3

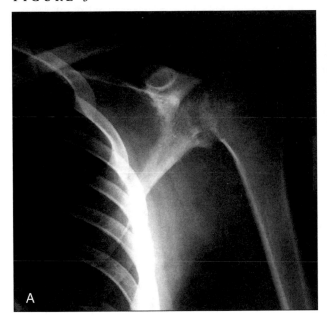

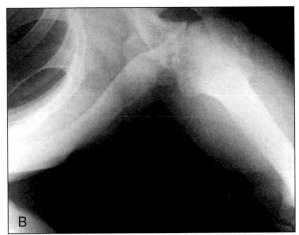

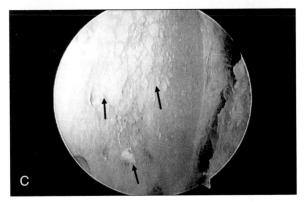

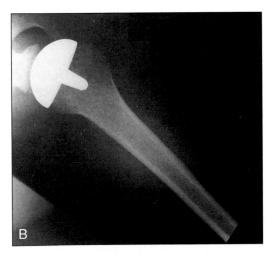

AP **(A)** and lateral **(B)** radiographs and arthroscopic photograph **(C)** of the shoulder of a 21-year-old man after thermal capsulorrhaphy with complete chondrolysis of the glenohumeral joint *(arrows)*.

FIGURE 4

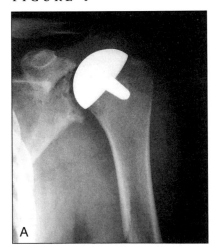

AP **(A)** and lateral **(B)** radiographs of humeral resurfacing combined with an interpositional lateral meniscal allograft as a salvage procedure for complete glenohumeral chondrolysis.

FIGURE 5

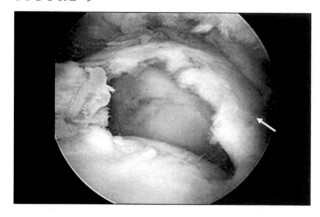

Failed arthroscopic rotator cuff repair *(arrow)* with suture pullout and breakage.

als with active spondylitis or a profile consistent with hypertrophic pulmonary osteoarthropathy (ie, obese, smoking, male laborers with a history of chronic pulmonary disease).[78]

Arthroscopic SAD for impingement produces results comparable with open procedures, mostly for symptomatic stage I and II lesions that have failed nonsurgical treatment. Failure rates of SAD have varied from 5% to 21%; most failures result from persistent uncorrected acromioclavicular (AC)[2] joint pain, inadequate decompression, or a coexisting rotator cuff tear.[4,36,49,53,82] Known complication rates are low (1% to 8%), and specific examples include instrument breakage (particularly burrs), transient neurapraxias, and excessive intraoperative bleeding.[1,2,4,34,36,49,82] Acromial fracture may result from overaggressive burr resection.[6,8,77]

Recognizing the role that the AC joint may play in a patient with subacromial pathology is also important. Arthritic AC joints may have too much or too little distal clavicle removed in conjunction with an acromioplasty; ideal management of the inferior AC osteophyte remains controversial, and violation of the AC joint during acromioplasty can be problematic.[6,83,84] Failure to completely remove the distal clavicle when indicated can lead to recurrent pain and failure.

Arthroscopic Rotator Cuff Repair

Complications, distinct from failures, are not very common in arthroscopic rotator cuff repair. Loose hardware is an infrequent but nonetheless recognized complica-

tion. Bioabsorbable tacks have had a steep learning curve and associated complication rate, much like the process of mastering arthroscopic knot tying for anatomic restoration of the rotator cuff. Weber and associates[8] reported that the complications and failures of arthroscopic rotator cuff repair mirror those of arthroscopic acromioplasty in that they are most likely multifactorial (Figure 5).

SUMMARY

Awareness of potential complications as discussed above is the most significant factor in prevention of complications associated with arthroscopic shoulder surgery. Recognition and proper management of complications associated with arthroscopic shoulder procedures is essential to obtaining optimal patient outcomes.

REFERENCES

1. Committee on Complications of the Arthroscopy Association of North America: Complications in arthroscopy: The knee and other joints. *Arthroscopy* 1986;2:253-258.

2. Small N: Complications in arthroscopic surgery performed by experienced arthroscopists. *Arthroscopy* 1988;4:215-221.

3. Berjano P, Gonzalez BG, Olmedo JF, Perez-Espana LA, Munilla MG: Complications in arthroscopic shoulder surgery. *Arthroscopy* 1998;14:785-788.

4. Bigliani L, Flatow E, Deliz E: Complications of shoulder arthroscopy. *Orthop Rev* 1991;20:743-751.

5. McFarland E, O'Neill O, Hsu C: Complications of shoulder arthroscopy. *J South Orthop Assoc* 1997;6:190-196.

6. Shaffer B, Tibone J: Arthroscopic shoulder instability surgery: Complications. *Clin Sports Med* 1999;18:737-767.

7. Small N: Complications in arthroscopic surgery of the knee and shoulder. *Orthopedics* 1993;16:985-988.

8. Weber SC, Abrams JS, Nottage WM: Complications associated with arthroscopic shoulder surgery. *Arthroscopy* 2002;18:88-95.

9. Rupp S, Sell R, Muller B, Kohn D: Abstract: Complications after subacromial decompression. *Arthroscopy* 1998;14:445.

10. Curtis AS, Snyder SJ, Del Pizzo W, Friedman MJ, Ferkel RD, Karzal RP: Abstract: Complications of shoulder arthroscopy. *Arthroscopy* 1992;8:395.

11. Borgeat A, Bird P, Ekatodramis G, Dumont C: Tracheal compression caused by periarticular fluid accumula-

tion: A rare complication of shoulder surgery. *J Shoulder Elbow Surg* 2000;9:443-445.

12. Dietzel D, Ciullo J: Spontaneous pneumothorax after shoulder arthroscopy: A report of four cases. *Arthroscopy* 1996;12:99-102.

13. Karns J: Epinephrine-induced potentially lethal arrhythmia during arthroscopic shoulder surgery: A case report. *AANA J* 1999;67:419-421.

14. Anderson A, Alfrey D, Lipscomb AJ: Acute pulmonary edema, an unusual complication following arthroscopy: A report of three cases. *Arthroscopy* 1990;6:235-237.

15. Pitman MI, Nainzadeh N, Ergas E, Springer S: The use of somatosensory evoked potentials for detection of neuropraxia during shoulder arthroscopy. *Arthroscopy* 1988;4:250-255.

16. Klein A, France JC, Mutschler TA, Fu FH: Measurement of brachial plexus strain in arthroscopy of the shoulder. *Arthroscopy* 1987;3:45-52.

17. Johnson LL, Schneider DA, Austin MD, Goodman FG, Bullock JM, DeBruin JH: Two per cent glutaraldehyde: A disinfectant in arthroscopy and arthroscopic surgery. *J Bone Joint Surg Am* 1982;64:237-239.

18. D'Angelo G, Ogilvie-Harris D: Septic arthritis following arthroscopy, with cost/benefit analysis of antibiotic prophylaxis. *Arthroscopy* 1988;4:10-14.

19. Armstrong R, Bolding F: Septic arthritis after arthroscopy: The contributing roles of intraarticular steroids and environmental factors. *Am J Infect Control* 1994;22:16-18.

20. Lee H, Dewan N, Crosby L: Subcutaneous emphysema, pneumomediastinum, and potentially life-threatening tension pneumothorax: Pulmonary complications from arthroscopic shoulder decompression. *Chest* 1992;101:1265-1267.

21. Lau K: Pneumomediastinum caused by subcutaneous emphysema in the shoulder: A rare complication of arthroscopy. *Chest* 1993;103:1606-1607.

22. Hegde R, Avatgere R: Air embolism during anaesthesia for shoulder arthroscopy. *Br J Anaesth* 2000;85:926-927.

23. Grunwald J, Bauer G, Wruhs O: Fatal complication in arthroscopy in a gaseous medium. *Unfallchirurg* 1987;90:97.

24. Habegger R, Siebenmann R, Kieser C: Lethal air embolism during arthroscopy: A case report. *J Bone Joint Surg Br* 1989;71:314-316.

25. Faure E, Cook R, Miles D: Air embolism during anesthesia for shoulder arthroscopy. *Anesthesiology* 1998;89:805-806.

26. Burkhart S: Deep venous thrombosis after shoulder arthroscopy. *Arthroscopy* 1990;6:61-63.

27. Polzhofer G, Petersen W, Hassenpflug J: Thromboembolic complication after arthroscopic shoulder surgery. *Arthroscopy* 2003;19:E16-E19.

28. Liguori G, Kahn RL, Gordon J, Gordon MA, Urban MK: The use of metoprolol and glycopyrrolate to prevent hypotensive/bradycardic events during shoulder arthroscopy in the sitting position under interscalene block. *Anesth Analg* 1998;87:1320-1325.

29. Andrews J, Carson WJ, Ortega K: Arthroscopy of the shoulder: Technique and normal anatomy. *Am J Sports Med* 1984;12:1-7.

30. Matthews L, Zarins B, Michael RH, Helfet DL: Anterior portal selection for shoulder arthroscopy. *Arthroscopy* 1985;1:33-39.

31. Detrisac D, Johnson L: *Arthroscopic Shoulder Anatomy: Pathologic and Surgical Implications.* Thorofare, NJ, Slack, 1986.

32. Flatow E, Bigliani L, April E: An anatomic study of the musculocutaneous nerve and its relationship to the coracoid process. *Clin Orthop Relat Res* 1989;244:166-171.

33. Davidson P, Tibone J: Anterior-inferior (5 o'clock) portal for shoulder arthroscopy. *Arthroscopy* 1995;11:519-525.

34. Ogilvie-Harris D, Wiley A: Arthroscopic surgery of the shoulder: A general appraisal. *J Bone Joint Surg Br* 1986;68:201-207.

35. Hawkins R: Arthroscopic stapling repair for shoulder instability: A retrospective study of 50 cases. *Arthroscopy* 1989;5:122-128.

36. Altchek D: Arthroscopic acromioplasty: Technique and results. *J Bone Joint Surg Am* 1990;72:1198-1207.

37. Jensen K, Werther K, Stryger V, Schultz K, Falkenberg B: Arthroscopic shoulder surgery with epinephrine saline irrigation. *Arthroscopy* 2001;17:578-581.

38. Morrison D, Schaefer R, Friedman R: The relationship between subacromial space pressure, blood pressure, and visual clarity during arthroscopic subacromial decompression. *Arthroscopy* 1995;11:557-560.

39. Burkhart S, Barnett C, Snyder S: Transient postoperative blindness as a possible effect of glycine toxicity. *Arthroscopy* 1990;6:112-114.

40. Ogilvie-Harris D, Boynton E: Arthroscopic acromioplasty: Extravasation of fluid into the deltoid muscle. *Arthroscopy* 1990;6:52-54.

41. Lee Y, Cohn L, Tooke S: Intramuscular deltoid pressure during shoulder arthroscopy. *Arthroscopy* 1989;5:209-212.

42. Yamaguchi K, Levine WN, Marra G, Galatz LM, Klepps S, Flatow EL: Transitioning to arthroscopic rotator cuff repair: The pros and cons. *Instr Course Lect* 2003;52:81-92.

43. Hynson JM, Tung A, Guevara JE, Katz JA, Glick JM, Shapiro WA: Complete airway obstruction during arthroscopic shoulder surgery. *Anesth Analg* 1993;76: 875-878.

44. Cameron S: Venous pseudoaneurysm as a complication of shoulder arthroscopy. *J Shoulder Elbow Surg* 1996;5:404-406.

45. Segmuller H, Alfred SP, Zilio G, Saies AD, Hayes MG: Cutaneous nerve lesions of the shoulder and arm after arthroscopic shoulder surgery. *J Shoulder Elbow Surg* 1995;4:254-258.

46. Skyhar MJ, Altchek DW, Warren RF, Wickiewicz TL, O'Brien SJ: Shoulder arthroscopy with the patient in the beach-chair position. *Arthroscopy* 1988;4:256-259.

47. Nottage W: Arthroscopic portals: Anatomy at risk. *Orthop Clin North Am* 1993;24:19-26.

48. Rodeo S, Forster R, Weiland A: Neurological complications due to arthroscopy. *J Bone Joint Surg Am* 1993;75:917-926.

49. Ellman H: Arthroscopic subacromial decompression: Analysis of one- to three-year results. *Arthroscopy* 1987;3:173-181.

50. Abstracts: Annual meeting of the AANA (Arthroscopy Association of North America). Boston, Massachusetts, April 10-13, 1985. *Arthoscopy* 1985;1:142-151.

51. Mullins R, Drez DJ, Cooper J: Hypoglossal nerve palsy after arthroscopy of the shoulder and open operation with the patient in the beach-chair position: A case report. *J Bone Joint Surg Am* 1992;74:137-139.

52. Mohammed K, Hayes M, Saies A: Unusual complications of shoulder arthroscopy. *J Shoulder Elbow Surg* 2000;9:350-353.

53. Norwood L, Fowler H: Rotator cuff tears: A shoulder arthroscopy complication. *Am J Sports Med* 1989;17: 837-841.

54. Souryal T, Baker C: Anatomy of the supraclavicular fossa portal in shoulder arthroscopy. *Arthroscopy* 1990;6:297-300.

55. Bonsell S: Detached deltoid during arthroscopic subacromial decompression. Arthroscopy 2000;16:745-748.

56. Mormino M, Gross R, McCarthy J: Captured shoulder: A complication of rotator cuff surgery. *Arthroscopy* 1996;12:457-461.

57. Warner JJ, Allen AA, Marks PH, Wong P: Arthroscopic release of postoperative capsular contracture of the shoulder. *J Bone Joint Surg Am* 1997;79:1151-1158.

58. Rockwood CA Jr: Shoulder arthroscopy. *J Bone Joint Surg Am* 1988;70:639-640.

59. Muller D, Landsiedl F: Abstract: Arthroscopy of the shoulder joint: A minimal invasive and harmless procedure? *Arthroscopy* 2000;16:425.

60. Moran M, Warren R: Development of a synovial cyst after arthroscopy of the shoulder: A brief note. *J Bone Joint Surg Am* 1989;71:127-129.

61. Matthews LS, Vetter WL, Oweida SJ, Spearman J, Helfet DL: Arthroscopic staple capsulorrhaphy for recurrent anterior shoulder instability. *Arthroscopy* 1988;4:106-111.

62. Ellman H: Arthroscopic treatment of impingement of the shoulder. *Instr Course Lect* 1989;38:177-185.

63. Morgan C, Bodenstab A: Arthroscopic Bankart suture repair: Technique and early results. *Arthroscopy* 1987;3:111-122.

64. Landsiedl F: Arthroscopic therapy of recurrent anterior luxation of the shoulder by capsular repair. *Arthroscopy* 1992;8:296-304.

65. Goldberg B, Nirschl RP, McConnell JP, Pettrone FA: Arthroscopic transglenoid suture capsulolabral repairs: Preliminary results. *Am J Sports Med* 1993;21:656-664.

66. Bigliani LU, Dalsey RM, McCann PD, April EW: An anatomical study of the suprascapular nerve. *Arthroscopy* 1990;6:301-305.

67. Bryan W, Schauder K, Tullos H: The axillary nerve and its relationship to common sports medicine shoulder procedures. *Am J Sports Med* 1986;14:113-116.

68. Shea K, Lovallo J: Scapulothoracic penetration of a Beath pin: An unusual complication of arthroscopic Bankart suture repair. *Arthroscopy* 1991;7:115-117.

69. Burkart A, Imhoff A, Roscher E: Foreign-body reaction to the bioabsorbable suretac device. *Arthroscopy* 2000; 16:91-95.

70. Rhee Y, Lee DH, Chun IH, Bae SC: Glenohumeral arthropathy after arthroscopic anterior shoulder stabilization. *Arthroscopy* 2004;20:402-406.

71. Freehill M, Harms DJ, Huber SM, Atlihan D, Buss DD: Poly-L-lactic acid tack synovitis after arthroscopic stabilization of the shoulder. *Am J Sports Med* 2003;31:643-647.

72. Petty D, Jazrawi LM, Estrada LS, Andrews JR: Glenohumeral chondrolysis after shoulder arthroscopy: Case reports and review of the literature. *Am J Sports Med* 2004;32:509-515.

73. D'Alessandro DF, Bradley JP, Fleischli JE, Connor PM: Prospective evaluation of thermal capsulorrhaphy for shoulder instability: Indications and results, two- to five-year follow-up. *Am J Sports Med* 2004;32:21-33.

74. Wong K, Williams G: Complications of thermal capsulorrhaphy of the shoulder. *J Bone Joint Surg Am* 2001;83(suppl 2):151-155.

75. McFarland EG, Kim TK, Banchasuek P, McCarthy EF: Histologic evaluation of the shoulder capsule in normal shoulders, unstable shoulders, and after failed thermal capsulorrhaphy. *Am J Sports Med* 2002;30:636-642.

76. Hanypsiak BT, Faulks C, Fine K, Malin E, Shaffer B, Connell M: Rupture of the biceps tendon after arthroscopic thermal capsulorrhaphy. *Arthroscopy* 2004; 20(suppl 2):77-79.

77. Matthews L, Blue J: Arthroscopic subacromial decompression: Avoidance of complications and enhancement of results. *Instr Course Lect* 1998;47:29-33.

78. Berg E, Ciullo J, Oglesby J: Failure of arthroscopic decompression by subacromial heterotopic ossification causing recurrent impingement. *Arthroscopy* 1994;10:158-161.

79. Boynton M, Enders T: Severe heterotopic ossification after arthroscopic acromioplasty: A case report. *J Shoulder Elbow Surg* 1999;8:495-497.

80. Pouliart N, Casteleyn P: Vanishing distal clavicle after arthroscopic acromioplasty. *Arthroscopy* 2000;16:855-857.

81. Esch J: Arthroscopic subacromial decompression and postoperative management. *Orthop Clin North Am* 1993;24:161-171.

82. Gartsman G: Arthroscopic acromioplasty for lesions of the rotator cuff. *J Bone Joint Surg Am* 1990;72:169-180.

83. Fischer BW, Gross RM, McCarthy JA, Arroyo JS: Incidence of acromioclavicular joint complications after arthroscopic subacromial decompression. *Arthroscopy* 1999;15:241-248.

84. Barber FA: Coplaning of the acromioclavicular joint. *Arthroscopy* 2001;17:913-917.

INDEX

Keep informed on a broad range of topics

Four easy ways to order!

1. **PHONE** (credit card orders)
   AAOS toll-free **(800) 626-6726**
   Monday through Friday, 8:00 am
   to 5:00 pm, Central Time.
   Customers outside of the U.S.
   and Canada, call ++(847)
   823-7186. **Please mention
   priority code 1870.**

2. **FAX** your purchase order and /
   or completed order form and
   credit card information toll-free
   to **(800) 823-8025**.
   Customers outside of the U.S.
   and Canada, fax to ++(847)
   823-8025.

3. **ONLINE** (secure credit card
   orders) via the Academy's ecatalog
   at **www.aaos.org/products.**
   Search by topic or learning format.

4. **MAIL** your completed order
   form with check to **AAOS, P.O.
   Box 75838, Chicago, Illinois
   60675-5838** (please allow
   three to four weeks for delivery).
   Send credit card payment directly
   to **AAOS, 6300 N. River
   Road, Rosemont, Illinois
   60018-4262.** Prices are
   subject to change without notice.

Shipping and Handling

Order Amount	U.S. (UPS Ground)
Up to $75.00	**$7.95**
$75.01 to $100.00	**$9.95**
$100.01 to $200.00	**$13.95**
$200.01 or $250.00	**$16.95**
Over $250.00	**$19.95**
Canada residents add $10.00 surcharge to rates above	

☑ Yes! Send me the monographs I have indicated.

Item no.	Title	Price	AAOS Member Price	Resident/ Military Price	Quantity	Total
02-832	**NEW! Shoulder Arthroscopy** Theodore A. Blaine, MD, Editor	$50	$40	$40		
02-797	**NEW! Bone Graft Substitutes** Gary E. Friedlaender, MD, Henry J. Mankin, MD, and Victor M. Goldberg, MD, Editors	$50	$40	$40		
02-796	**NEW! Stiff Elbow** Jesse Jupiter, MD, Editor	$50	$40	$40		
02-795	**NEW! Complications in Orthopaedics: Spine Surgery** Raj Rao, MD, Editor	$50	$40	$40		
02-788	**Low Back Pain** Louis G. Jenis, MD, Editor	$50	$40	$40		
02-779	**Complications in Orthopaedics: Anterior Cruciate Ligament Surgery** Kevin B. Freedman, MD, MSCE, Editor	$50	$40	$40		
02-766	**Proximal Humerus Fractures** Michael A. Wirth, MD, Editor	$50	$40	$40		
02-765	**Complications in Orthopaedics: Distal Radius Fractures** Steven Friedman, MD, Editor	$50	$40	$40		
02-758	**Common Patellofemoral Problems** John P. Fulkerson, MD, Editor	$50	$40	$40		
02-713	**Neck Pain** Jeffrey Fischgrund, MD, Editor	$50	$40	$40		
02-714	**Adolescent Idiopathic Scoliosis** Peter Newton, MD, Editor	$50	$40	$40		
02-693	**Complications in Orthopaedics: Pediatric Upper Extremity Fractures** Charles Price, MD, Editor	$50	$40	$40		
02-692	**Complications in Orthopaedics: Tibial Shaft Fractures** William M. Ricci, MD, Editor	$50	$40	$40		
02-609	**Management of Osteoarthritis of the Knee** Freddie H. Fu, MD, and Bruce D. Browner, MD, Editors	$50	$40	$40		
02-579	**Revision Total Knee Arthroplasty** Leo A. Whiteside, MD, Editor	$50	$40	$40		
02-523	**Revision Total Hip Arthroplasty** Wayne G. Paprosky, MD, FACS, Editor	$50	$40	$40		
02-574	**Multiple Ligamentous Injuries of the Knee in the Athlete** Robert C. Schenck Jr., MD, Editor	$50	$40	$40		
02-413	**Arthroscopic Meniscal Repair** W. Dilworth Cannon Jr., MD, Editor	$50	$40	$40		
02-245	**The Female Athlete** Carol Teitz, MD	$50	$40	$40		
02-509	**Total Shoulder Arthroplasty** Lynn A. Crosby, MD, Editor	$50	$40	$40		

International customers: Email AAOS
Customer Service at **custserv@aaos.org** for
ordering information, including where to obtain
Academy products in your geographical area.

Subtotal	
Illinois purchasers add 9% sales tax	
Shipping and handling (see chart at left)	
Total	

Method of Payment

❑ Check or money order payable to AAOS enclosed (U.S. funds only)

❑ Purchase order enclosed (P.O.s will be accepted from institutions only)

❑ Visa   ❑ MasterCard   ❑ American Express

_____   _____
Card Number   Exp Date

_____
Signature

Ship to:

_____
Name   Academy ID Number

_____
Address

_____
City   State/Province   Zip/Postal Code

_____
Daytime Telephone   Fax Number

_____
Email

Subscribe and stay current on clinical issues and challenges!

Receive each new monograph <u>immediately upon publication</u> — about 5 per year — at a $5 discount from the list or member price.

❑ **Yes! I want to subscribe to the Monograph Series!**